S0-ACK-461

SURGICAL REPAIR AND RECONSTRUCTION IN RHEUMATOID DISEASE

SURGICAL REPAIR
AND RECONSTRUCTION
IN RHEUMATOID DISEASE

Alexander Benjamin MB, BS, FRCS

Orthopaedic Surgeon to Peace Memorial Hospital, Watford, Herts
West Herts Hospital, Hemel Hempstead, Herts
Honorary Lecturer, Postgraduate Institute of Orthopaedics, London

and

Basil Helal MB, BS, MCh(Orth), FRCS

Orthopaedic Surgeon to The London Hospital
Chase Farm Hospital, Enfield, Middlesex
Highlands Hospital, Winchmore Hill, London

A WILEY MEDICAL PUBLICATION

JOHN WILEY & SONS

New York · Chichester · Brisbane · Toronto

John Wiley and Sons Inc.,
605 Third Avenue, New York, NY 10016

First published 1980 by
The Macmillan Press Ltd
London and Basingstoke

© *1980 Alexander Benjamin and Basil Helal*

Printed in Great Britain

All rights reserved. No part of
this book may be reprinted, or reproduced
or utilized in any form or by any electronic,
mechanical or other means, now known or hereafter
invented, including photocopying and recording,
or in any information storage or retrieval system,
without permission in writing from the publisher.

British Library Cataloguing in Publication Data

Benjamin, Alexander
Surgical repair and reconstruction in
rheumatoid disease.
1. Rheumatoid arthritis – Surgery
I. Title   II. Helal, Basil
617′.472   RD686

ISBN 0–471–08291–0   LCCCN 80–50604

WE
346
B468s
1980

CONTENTS

64064

FOREWORD 1

Barbara M. Ansell, Clinical Research Centre, Division of Rheumatology Northwick Park.

Despite the cause, or causes, of rheumatoid disease still evading elucidation, the overall care of patients with this serious and potentially crippling illness has improved remarkably in the last two to three decades. This is partly due to the increased number of drugs available and a better understanding of how to use them, but particularly to the close collaboration of orthopaedic surgeons and physicians in attempting to minimise pain and disability not only through the appropriate use of drugs, but by the critical employment of recognised surgical techniques and the development of new ones.

Alec Benjamin and Basil Helal, who have extensive experience, open with general remarks on rheumatoid disease and the links with medical management, before discussing pre-operative assessment of patients and the main types of operative techniques that are available; chapters relating to specific joints or sites follow. This is a thoughtful and thought-provoking book which demonstrates critically the indications and outcome of the operations that are available. Perhaps even more important, it offers advice on the selection of the most suitable procedure for any given patient at a certain stage in the disease. At the present state of our knowledge the guidelines that these authors have tried to establish will be of great help to rheumatologists and orthopaedic surgeons alike. The development of improved techniques and the reappraisal of old ones will necessitate re-definition of indications for management. However, for many years to come this book will aid any team aiming to improve function and relieve pain through the surgical treatment of rheumatoid arthritis.

FOREWORD 2

Kauko Vainio, Heinola, Finland

Although surgery has blossomed over the past century, rheumatoid arthritis was until relatively recent times taboo for the surgeon with the exception of a few brave pioneers. The fear was that operation might cause an exacerbation of the disease and a more important factor was that co-operation between surgeons and rheumatologists was, at best, very poor. During the past 25 years the climate of opinion has changed completely. Surgery is now an'inseparable part of the overall treatment of rheumatoid disease and there is a close liaison between surgeon and rheumatologist.

The authors point out the fact that the surgeon and rheumatologist must be able to speak the same language. Thus, they start the book with a chapter on the pathology and medical management of the disease, not forgetting the important psychological factors. The chapter includes the latest knowledge on these subjects and will be of value to every surgeon.

Before discussing treatment of the individual joints the authors deal in general with the basic operations in rheumatoid arthritis, viz. synovectomy, osteotomy, arthroplasty and arthrodesis. They warn against over-enthusiasm in the use of prostheses and lay stress on the possible complications. They use osteotomies much more than many surgeons. This is an easy and inexpensive operation and if the results in suitable cases are comparable with those using expensive prostheses then the procedure should be used more. Multicentral research is necessary to elucidate this point.

In the chapters concerning interventions in different joints the authors present several new methods. These, as well as the old ones, are described sufficiently accurately to make it possible for every specialist to follow the techniques described which are clarified with numerous illustrations.

As an elderly surgeon who has spent his working life closely involved in the development of surgery of rheumatoid arthritis I welcome this new book with great pleasure.

PREFACE

This book draws largely on personal experience and is a practical guide to what we consider to be the best practice in the management of this difficult disease. We have been didactic in our presentation but are aware that other methods can have similar results. On controversial issues we have tried to present a reasoned synthesis of opinion, and whereas our own views occasionally conflict, we have found a degree of agreement perhaps unusual between two orthopaedic surgeons.

The seeds of this book were sown in 1970 at a meeting held to found the Rheumatoid Arthritis Surgical Society. The authors formed half of the quartet which founded the Society. Much of what we have learned has been gleaned at our meetings from fellow members, who, between them, represent a global opinion on this subject, for they include prominent rheumatological surgeons from Austria, Canada, Finland, Germany, Norway, Poland, Spain, Sweden, Switzerland and the United States of America.

Two of the members from Britain, George Arden and Barbara Ansell, have combined their unique experience into a book, *The Surgical Management of Juvenile Chronic Polyarthritis*, published by Academic Press Ltd. We have therefore deliberately avoided touching upon this topic and trust that the two books will complement each other.

We appreciate the tolerance of our wives, Stella and Bobbie, and of our children, and apologise for the many 'lost' evenings and weekends. We also greatly appreciate the remarkable patience of our secretaries, Bobbie Benjamin and Jenny Parke.

We are most grateful to the many surgeons and physicians and others who have kindly provided us with photographic material. They are individually acknowledged and we beg forgiveness of anyone we have omitted to mention.

We are indebted to John Collins of the Royal National Orthopaedic Hospital, to Martin Moor of Enfield District Hospital, to Ray Ruddick of the London Hospital and to Sidney Berlanney for photography, and to John Waterhouse for the art work.

As script readers we were most fortunate in having John Kirkup, Michael Salz and Michael Sullivan. Their wisdom and advice has been valuable beyond measure.

The co-operation of Macmillan Press Ltd has been exemplary and we are indebted to them for the smooth and rapid passage to publication.

We are honoured that Kauko Vainio and Barbara Ansell, who are, respectively, two of the most outstanding contributors to the surgical and medical aspects of rheumatology, have compiled the forewords.

Finally we take this opportunity to thank our teachers, many of whom are from our medical school, The London Hospital.

A. B.
B. H.

1

GENERAL CONSIDERATIONS

Rheumatoid arthritis may be a relatively modern disease, for there is no good archaeological evidence for its existence in ancient times (Caughey, 1974). Diseases which are recognised as rheumatic in type have been described since 500 BC. The term 'rheumatism' is said to have been used by Galen and Dioscorides in the first century AD. In 1857 Robert Adams in Dublin coined the term 'chronic rheumatic arthritis' and accurately illustrated the surgical pathology of the common manifestations of chronic joint disease. Sir Alfred Baring Garrod first proposed the term 'rheumatoid arthritis' in 1858. Currently, about 2 per cent of the population (in the western hemisphere) are affected by the disease and it affects three times as many women as men (see p. 217).

PATHOLOGY

The pathology is characterised by three principal features:

(1) The rheumatoid nodule is a type of granulomatous lesion consisting of an area of collagen necrosis with lymphoid infiltration; any contained vessels exhibit vasculitis.

(2) The synovitis is characterised by lymphoid infiltration, multiplication of surface cells, and fibrin formation, the contained vessels show vasculitis.

(3) The vasculitis, which can involve vessels of all calibres, is responsible for many of the extra-articular manifestations of the disease.

The disease results in synovial hypertrophy affecting joints, tendon sheaths and bursae but can affect all systems; systemic features are associated with increased likelihood of early death. Ten per cent of patients with systemic manifestations die from intercurrent infection. The systemic features include weight loss, lymphadenopathy, infections and osteoporosis which may be associated with stress fractures. Anaemia may be of the iron deficiency or the normocytic type, and the heart may be involved by myocarditis, coronary arteritis, pericarditis and valve granulomata. The lungs can be affected by rheumatoid nodules, fibrosing rheumatoid pneumoconiosis (Caplan's syndrome) and bronchiolitis. When there is liver and spleen enlargement combined with neutropenia, it is called Felty's syndrome.

Peripheral vasculitis and endarteritis may produce lesions ranging from skin ulcers to frank gangrene. When larger vessels are involved, cardiovascular catastrophes and mesenteric artery thromboses with bowel gangrene can occur. When medium-bore vessels are involved, ischaemia of nerves and renal tissues may supervene.

The eye may be involved by keratoconjunctivitis sicca (Sjögren's syndrome), and iridocyclitis. Amyloidosis is now largely the result of rheumatoid disease.

The aetiology and incidence are discussed in chapters 2 and 16.

DIAGNOSIS

Rheumatoid disease is diagnosed by a characteristic pattern of connective tissue abnormality. There are many variations within this pattern and consequently the list of named diseases is long and still growing.

We are concerned with those aspects of rheumatoid diseases of interest to the surgeon and will only mention particular diagnostic subdivisions when these are of surgical significance. The American Rheumatism Association has published criteria for the diagnosis of Classical, Definite, Probable and Possible Rheumatoid Arthritis (table 1.1).

The ease of diagnosis varies from cases in which it is self-evident to those where the diagnosis remains in doubt despite careful investigation. Monarticular arthritis may be the only manifestation and generalised rheumatoid disease may not develop for many years. In the absence of positive serological findings (IgM rheumatoid factor) the development of other stigmata of the disease often makes the diagnosis possible. An account of seronegative disease is given by Wright and Moll in their book *Seronegative Polyarthritis* (Wright and Moll, 1976).

A full history is essential and the surgeon must ask particular questions not necessarily directly related to the joint or part under consideration. It is important, for example, to ask whether or not there is morning stiffness.

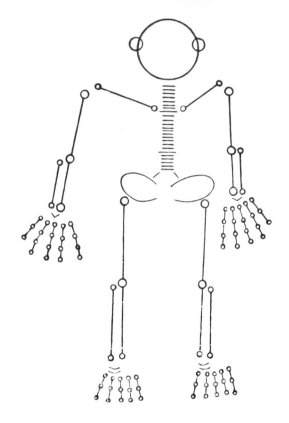

Figure 1.1 Rubber stamp for use in notes to record the pattern of joint involvement

The structures examined by the surgeon must include the overlying skin, subcutaneous tissues and adjacent muscles. The general condition of the patient is observed—in particular, the presence of wasting and anaemia. The pattern of joint involvement is relevant and is best recorded on a skeletal outline in the notes, each affected joint being ringed (figure 1.1). Some conditions usually treated individually may herald the onset of rheumatoid disease. Thus multiple trigger fingers may be the presenting feature of rheumatoid disease and a biopsy specimen of the synovium should be taken if a tendon sheath is incised. Intermetatarsal bursae if removed should always be examined microscopically, as these also may be the first manifestations of rheumatoid disease. Plantar fasciitis and ligament calcium deposition at the shoulder or elsewhere (figure 1.2) may similarly herald rheumatoid disease.

TABLE 1.1 DIAGNOSTIC CRITERIA FOR RHEUMATOID ARTHRITIS

Classical Rheumatoid Arthritis

This is to be diagnosed only if at least seven of the following criteria are present and if the total duration of joint symptoms including swelling has been continuous for at least 6 weeks:

(1) Morning stiffness (1 hour or more).
(2) Pain on motion or tenderness in at least one joint.
(3) Swelling (soft tissue thickening or fluid—not bony overgrowth alone) in at least one joint continuously for not less than 6 weeks.
(4) Swelling of at least one other joint (any interval free of joint symptoms between the two joint involvements may not be more than 3 months).
(5) Symmetrical joint swelling with simultaneous involvement of the same joint on both sides of the body (bilateral involvement of proximal interphalangeal, metacarpophalangeal or metatarsophalangeal joints is acceptable without absolute symmetry). Distal interphalangeal joint involvement will not satisfy this criterion.
(6) Subcutaneous nodules over bony prominences, on extensor surfaces or in juxta-articular regions.
(7) X-ray changes typical of rheumatoid arthritis (which must include at least bony decalcification localised to, or greatest around, the involved joints and not just degenerative changes). However, degenerative changes do not exclude the diagnosis of rheumatoid arthritis.
(8) Positive sheep cell agglutination test. (Any modification will suffice that does not give more than 5 per cent of positive results in non-rheumatoid control subjects.)
(9) Poor mucin precipitate from synovial fluid (with shreds and cloudy solution).

(10) Characteristic histological changes in synovial membrane with three or more of the following: marked villous hypertrophy; proliferation of superficial synovial cells often with palisading; marked infiltration of chronic inflammatory cells (lymphocytes or plasma cells predominating) with tendency to form 'lymphoid nodules'; deposition of compact fibrin, either on the surface or interstitially; foci of cell necrosis.
(11) Characteristic histological changes in nodules showing granulomatous foci with central zones of cell necrosis, surrounded by proliferated fixed cells, and peripheral fibrosis and chronic inflammatory cell infiltration, predominantly perivascular.

Definite Rheumatoid Arthritis

This diagnosis calls for at least five of the above criteria with a total duration of joint symptoms, including swelling, for a continuous period of at least 6 weeks.

Probable Rheumatoid Arthritis

This diagnosis requires at least three of the above criteria and a total duration of joint symptoms of at least 4 weeks.

Possible Rheumatoid Arthritis

This diagnosis requires two of the following criteria and total duration of joint symptoms of at least 3 weeks:

(1) Morning stiffness.
(2) Tenderness or pain on motion with history of recurrence or persistence for 3 weeks.
(3) History of observation of joint swelling.
(4) Subcutaneous nodules.
(5) Elevated sedimentation rate or increased C-reactive protein.
(6) Iritis.

COURSE OF THE DISEASE

Rheumatoid disease is characterised by exacerbations and remissions and may advance until the patient is confined to bed or chair. Pregnancy, a surgical operation or an injury may initiate an exacerbation with consequent deterioration. Nevertheless the disease may wane spontaneously at any time and there is sound basis for hope and encouragement rather than despair.

SURGICAL REGIMEN

Diseased joints must not be regarded in isolation, but must be considered in relation to the patient as a whole. Fitness for surgery is carefully assessed and anaemia is corrected. The planned surgical regimen must offer a reasonable chance that the patient will be better as the result of the surgery than if left untreated. This may appear obvious but sometimes surgical enthusiasm has to be

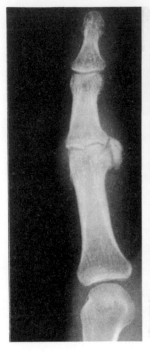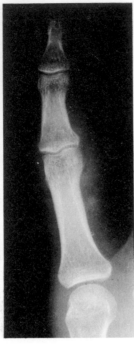

Figure 1.2 Acute painful calcium salt deposition in the collateral ligament of a proximal interphalangeal joint before and after curettage

disease. The capacity to walk may depend on the ability to use crutches or other walking-aids. When upper limb surgery is considered, thought must be given to its effect on the ability or potential ability to use such aids, and when lower limb surgery is considered, to its effect on the upper limbs in both the present and the future. The patient with a stiff knee may depend on good upper limbs to rise from a chair. Should the upper limbs deteriorate, considerable disability may result from a knee arthrodesis performed years previously.

INDICATIONS FOR SURGERY

(1) To relieve pain.
(2) To improve and maintain function.
(3) To prevent deformity.
(4) To correct deformity and instability.
(5) To attempt to arrest the disease.
(6) To improve appearance.

Pain unrelieved by conservative measures is the most important indication for surgery. Surgery which corrects deformity may impair function; all considerations other than pain should be subservient to function. Many deformed hands have been corrected surgically when to the dismay of the patient the ability to knit, sew and perhaps lift a cup of tea is lost. Pain relief may be achieved by synovectomy, osteotomy, arthrodesis or arthroplasty. Function may be improved by relief of pain or by the stabilisation of an unstable joint by osteotomy, arthrodesis or prosthetic replacement.

Deformity may be prevented and corrected by the procedures mentioned or by tendon realignment. In the early stage of a deformity such as ulnar drift of the fingers, surgery may be justified to prevent the almost inevitable advance of the condition. Radial deviation at the wrist predisposes to the development of ulnar deviation of the fingers resulting in the Z deformity. Osteotomy of the radius, removing an ulnar-based wedge, may thus prevent this deformity (Davison and Caird, 1976). Preventive surgery is not to be undertaken lightly, as ulnar deviation of the fingers is painless and often does not significantly impair function. It was thought that synovectomy

curbed. It may emanate from the physician, and a recommendation for surgery by him and its rejection by his surgical colleague may indicate a good working relationship between them. If the surgical procedure fails, retrieval of the situation must be possible—for example, a total knee replacement is acceptable only if sufficient bone is left to permit arthrodesis should the prosthesis have to be discarded. When several surgical procedures are indicated, the disadvantage of simultaneous multiple operations has to be balanced against life expectancy. Surgery on several joints under one anaesthetic may be indicated in rheumatoid disease, whereas only one such procedure would be contemplated in a non-rheumatoid patient. The length of the regimen of surgical treatment needs to be significantly shorter than the life expectancy.

Before operation it is incumbent upon the surgeon to assess the state of the other joints affected and to look into the likely progress of the

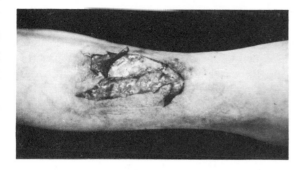

Figure 1.3 An area of skin over the tibia wiped off by careless handling of a patient who was on long-term steroid therapy

prevents further rheumatoid damage to a joint; this may be so but not all evidence supports this contention. Tendon decompression does prevent tendon rupture and synovectomy is probably unnecessary, but the temptation to remove the proliferative rheumatoid synovium is usually too great for the surgeon to resist (Savill, 1972). Appearance is improved by correction of deformity and the removal of rheumatoid nodules. It is particularly on the fingers that the removal of these nodules for cosmetic reasons is appreciated.

ANAESTHESIA AND SPECIAL CARE DURING SURGERY

Owing to skin fragility, diminished subcutaneous fat, vasculitis, porosity of bone and loss of ligament strength, particular care has to be taken in handling the patient with rheumatoid disease. Finger pressure on the abnormal skin may leave prints and cause bruising or separation of skin from the deep fascia, as also may a roughly applied Esmarch bandage. The skin over the subcutaneous border of the tibia is most susceptible (figure 1.3) but all areas require care, including the facial skin, which may be damaged by the anaesthetist's fingers. This problem is exaggerated by long-term steroid therapy. Foam bandages may be applied to protect the shins and may also be used to relieve pressure on heels and elbows. The cervical spine requires particular care as

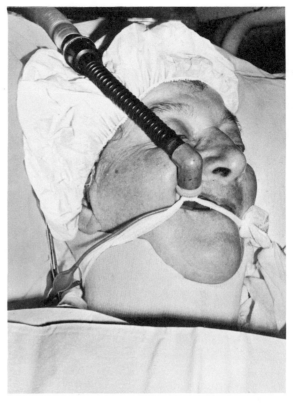

Figure 1.4 A soft cervical collar worn by rheumatoid patients in the operating theatre reminds staff that special care is required owing to soft tissue and bone fragility

instability may have been caused by destruction of bone and ligaments by rheumatoid disease. This process may be silent and impossible to diagnose on physical examination. There is danger of vertebral subluxation and transection of the cervical cord, particularly when the head is manipulated during laryngeal intubation. An X-ray of the cervical spine is advisable prior to a general anaesthetic and a soft collar worn during surgery reminds all staff in the theatre that particular care should be taken not to strain the neck (figure 1.4). Ankylosis of the temporomandibular joints, cricoarytenoid arthritis, as well as neck deformity or instability may make laryngeal intubation difficult and the use of ketamine or spinal anaesthesia without intubation may be necessary. Care must be taken with the choice of anaesthetic agent, as patients with rheumatoid disease are liable to

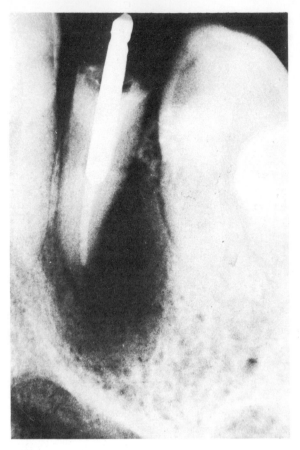

Figure 1.5 Silent root abscess in rheumatoid disease associated with a previous root filling

the aspirate subjected to microscopy and culture whenever infection is considered possible. Other signs of infection such as a raised ESR and white blood cell count may be absent. In the past 18 years 100 cases of septic arthritis in rheumatoid disease have been reported, of which one-third died (Goldenberg *et al.*, 1975). Early diagnosis and treatment by systemic antibiotics and adequate drainage improves the prognosis. Drainage by arthrotomy and thorough irrigation at operation followed for 24 h by through and through irrigations is advised (Gristina, Rovere and Shoje, 1974). Intercurrent infection is to be treated with care and antibiotics are indicated more frequently than in non-rheumatoid disease. The presence of a prosthetic joint is a particular indication for antibiotics should there be infection anywhere in the body, and antibiotic cover is advised whenever a tooth is extracted. Dental root fillings are contraindicated in rheumatoid disease because an abscess associated with such a root is likely to be silent and possibly become a source of bacteraemia, menacing a prosthesis and putting life itself at risk (figure 1.5).

CORTICOSTEROIDS

The stress of surgery or anaesthesia in a patient who is on long-term corticosteroid therapy or who has had such therapy recently may precipitate an Addisonian hypotensive crisis. Staff should be warned, the patient closely monitored and a syringe containing hydrocortisone kept at the bedside to use in emergency. It is customary in some units to give corticosteroid cover during surgery, and whereas this may be advisable, it does not exclude the possibility of a hypotensive crisis. Corticosteroid cover should not lull the staff into a false sense of security and they should remain alert to this rare but potentially fatal complication (Plumpton, Besser and Cole, 1969).

develop sensitivity; thus repeated halothane administration may induce liver damage.

BACTERIAL INFECTION AND SEPTIC ARTHRITIS

Patients with rheumatoid arthritis are particularly susceptible to bacterial infection. The morbidity from such infection has been reduced since the introduction of antibiotics but is increased in those patients on corticosteroids. Rheumatoid patients with bacterial infection tend to develop septic arthritis (Kellgren, 1958). The diagnosis between a rheumatoid exacerbation and a septic arthritis may be difficult. The possibility must be continually kept in mind and the joint aspirated and

BED REST

Prolonged bed rest is detrimental, whereas a short period of rest is often excellent therapy. The

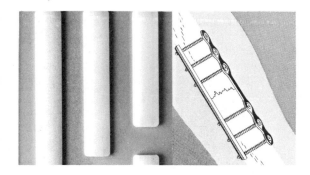

Figure 1.6 High-density polyethylene plates (Gallannaugh) may be used alone or in combination with standard bone plates (Zimmer (GB) Ltd)

diseased joints stiffen and the patient who is just able to care for herself, being able to get out of bed, dress and walk, may become a dependent invalid after only a few weeks in bed. A fracture of the femoral shaft which may be treated by traction in other patients is better treated by internal fixation in the rheumatoid patient to allow early walking and avoid the ill-effects of prolonged rest. Porotic rheumatoid bones do not afford good fixation for plates and screws and may require additional external splintage. A high-density polyethylene plate in combination with a metal plate is suitable for the internal fixation of porotic bone (Gallan-

Figure 1.7 The Chichester instrumentation. The nylon straps are self-locking and will not loosen. The studs on the nylon straps prevent obstruction of the blood vessels (A. Partridge)

naugh, 1975; figure 1.6). The Chichester instrumentation now being developed shows promise (chapter 13; figures 1.7–1.8) (Partridge, 1977).

PSYCHOLOGICAL FACTORS

Psychological factors influence the onset and course of rheumatoid disease: personality factors seem to play a part in its development and stress is related to the onset of the disease (Solomon, 1965). Rheumatoid females show more self-sacrifice, subservience, depression and sensitivity to the anger of others when compared with their healthy sisters. There is evidence that stress may influence the immune response, possibly by increase of adrenal cortical hormones, and that the immune response may be regulated by the hypothalamus. The somatic effects of stress were described by Hans Selye in 1950. Psychological measurements such as those used in MMPI (Minnesota Multiphasic Personality Inventory) (McKinley and Hathaway, 1943) ratings have not yet been developed sufficiently for routine use. Psychometric studies are likely to become a valuable tool in the assessment of the rheumatoid patient and thus assist the surgeon in his decisions. The depressed rheumatoid patient is a poor candidate for surgery, and unless the depression is clearly ex-

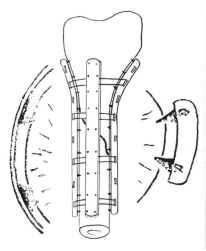
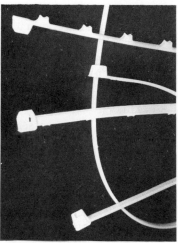
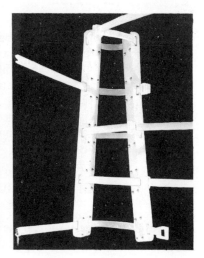

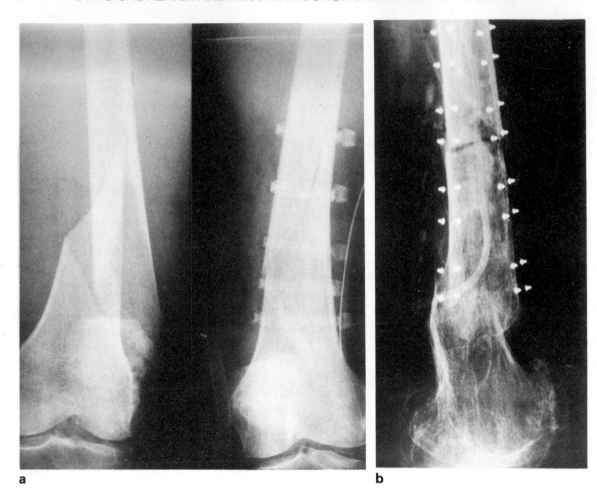

a   b

Figure 1.8 Radiographs of femoral fractures internally fixed with Chichester straps only (a) and following a second fracture, studded plates with straps (b) (N. Roles)

ogenous, the result is likely to be bad, whatever the procedure. The progress of rheumatoid disease is influenced by psychological problems. A patient who suffered from both rheumatoid disease and asthma was observed for 25 years. During times of psychological stress she developed either an episode of asthma or an exacerbation of her generalised rheumatoid disease.

RESULTS OF SURGERY

The result of surgery on the rheumatoid patient depends not only on the local pathology and the technical procedure undertaken, but also on the state of the systemic disease. A depressed patient who is sero-positive with a high ESR, LE cells and advancing disease and is on corticosteroid therapy is likely to have a worse result following surgery than a psychologically well-balanced patient who is sero-negative with quiescent disease.

The correct surgical procedure for a patient with rheumatoid disease depends on broad consideration of the available data by the rheumatologist and the surgeon. The selection of the procedure and its application at the appropriate stage has considerable bearing on subsequent success or failure.

REFERENCES

Caughey, D. E. (1974). The Arthritis of Constantine IX. *Ann. Rheum. Dis.*, **33** 77

Davison, E. P. and Caird, D. M. (1976). Osteotomy of the radius in rheumatoid disease, *Br. Orth. Ass.*, Spring Meeting

Diagnostic Criteria for Rheumatoid Arthritis (1959). *Ann. Rheum. Dis.*, **18**, 49–51

Gallannaugh, S. C. (1975). High density polyethylene plate for fracture fixation in the elderly, *Br. Med. J.*, December 6, 560–561

Garrod, A. B. (1876). *A Treatise on Gout and Rheumatic Gout (Rheumatoid Arthritis)*, 3rd edn, Longmans Green, London, p. 498

Goldenberg, D. L., Brandt, K. D., Cohen, A. S. and Cathcart, E. S. (1975). Treatment of septic arthritis: comparison of needle aspiration and surgery as initial modes of joint drainage. *Arth. Rheum.*, **18**, 83

Gristina, A. G., Rovere, G. D. and Shoje, H. (1974). *J. Bone Jt Surg.*, **56A,** 1180

Kellgren, J. H. (1958). *Br. Med. J.*, **1**, 1193

McKinley, J. C. and Hathaway, S. R. (1943). The identification and measurement of the psychoneuroses in medical practice, *J. Am. Med. Ass.*, **122,** 161–167

Partridge, A. (1977). Nylon plates and straps for internal fixation of osteoporotic bone. *Lancet*, April 9, 808

Plumpton, F. S., Besser, G. M. and Cole, P. V. (1969). Corticosteroid treatment and surgery. *Anaesthesia*, **24** (1), 3–18.

Savill, D. L. (1972). Surgery of the rheumatoid hand. *J. Bone Jt Surg.*, **54B,** 559

Selye, H. (1950). *The Physiology and Pathology of Exposure to Stress*, ACTA Inc., Montreal

Solomon, G. F. (1965). The relationship of personality to the presence of rheumatoid factor in asymptomatic relatives of patients with rheumatoid arthritis. *Psychosom. Med.*, **27**, 350

Wright, V. and Moll, J. M. H. (1976). *Seronegative Polyarthritis*, North-Holland, Amsterdam

2

THE LINK WITH MEDICAL MANAGEMENT

The medical and surgical care of the patient with rheumatoid disease is best achieved by consultation between physician and surgeon in a combined out-patient clinic. As on average two new joints are affected by the rheumatoid process every 3 years, the patient requires constant psychological, as well as medical and surgical, support. And whereas it is not helpful to offer false hope, it is harmful to say to the patient: 'Nothing can be done for you'. We are able to cure few, but can help many and give comfort to all. In the combined clinic the physician, surgeon and social workers also have the opportunity to learn much of the patient's home and social environment. In treating rheumatoid disease it is said to be better to know the patient who has a disability rather than to know the disability which the patient has (Swanson, 1977). We believe it is best to know both.

ANAEMIA

Anaemia is a common feature of the disease and subclinical gastro-intestinal haemorrhage from salicylates and other anti-inflammatory drugs may aggravate it. One should distinguish between the normochromic normocytic anaemia which is part of the disease and the iron deficiency anaemia which is the result of therapy; therapy for the latter will raise the haemoglobin up to a level consistent with the severity of the disease activity but no more. The iron may have to be administered by the intramuscular route as there is poor absorption of iron in the active disease and if penicillamine is being administered it has a chelating effect. In resistant anaemia blood transfusion may be indicated, and in the presence of hypersplenism in Felty's syndrome splenectomy may be beneficial.

REST

Rest is an important factor in management and bed rest in hospital in the acute phase may be therapeutic provided it is not prolonged. The acutely inflamed joints benefit and the temporary removal of the patient from the home environment may reduce psychological stress. Extended periods of rest are harmful, and treatment is instituted to strengthen muscles and prevent the development of deformity. Splints should be used

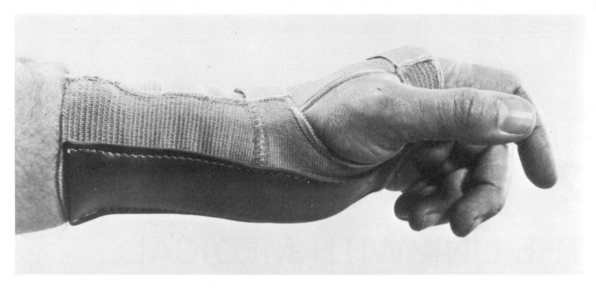

Figure 2.1 Futuro wrist splint (Seton Products)

to control deforming forces and rest an inflamed joint while enabling the other joints to be exercised.

Joints may be splinted with plaster of Paris slabs or specially designed supports. A back slab for the knee bandaged on at night helps prevent the development of flexion deformity and a right-angle splint for the ankle helps prevent an equinus deformity. A wrist splint reduces pain and increases stability, so improving the grip and mobility of the hand (figure 2.1). Flexion deformity at the wrist can be manipulated into extension under anaesthetic and held in this position for several weeks in plaster; treated thus, it may pass through a painful phase without the development of a fixed deformity and so avoid surgical intervention.

PHYSIOTHERAPY

Physiotherapy helps to reduce pain and swelling, to prevent and diminish deformity, to strengthen weak muscles and to assist rehabilitation. Active exercise may be prescribed provided joint pain is not increased. Isometric exercises with the knee extended strengthen the quadriceps muscle without aggravating knee arthritis, whereas exercises with knee flexion increase pain in the presence of patellofemoral disease.

Passive movement of joints as advised by Menell and Maitland (Mennell, 1960; Maitland, 1970) is of great value in the hands of a skilled physiotherapist. Passive joint movement in unskilled hands may cause damage and is especially harmful for the shoulder and elbow. Menell manipulations stretch joint capsules to the limit of the pain-free range. Traction is applied and the joint is moved passively through an arc frequently not within its normal range of active movement. For example, interphalangeal joints are rocked from side to side and the shoulder is manipulated by grasping the arm just below the axilla and moving the head of the humerus across the plane of the glenoid. Maitland manipulations are small strong oscillatory movements applicable to the spinal facet joints. Pain, swelling and muscle spasm are relieved by the local application of heat and sometimes cold, the more effective of these being chosen by trial and error. Employed at the beginning of each session of physiotherapy, these measures facilitate subsequent exercises which otherwise might be limited by pain, swelling and muscle spasm.

LOCAL INJECTION

Local injection of steroid, local anaesthetic and hyalase into painful nodules, ligaments or periarticular tissues as well as intra-articularly, often gives lasting pain relief. The immediate effect of the local anaesthetic will indicate whether the steroid is in the correct site. An aseptic technique is advised with physician or surgeon masked and wearing sterile gloves and the part cleaned and draped with sterile towels. This is considered an impractical counsel of perfection by some, but it is nevertheless desirable in intra-articular injections. The more successful the intra-articular pain relief the more likely it is that destructive degenerative changes will follow (figure 2.10a and b). Careful judgement is necessary to balance this risk against the benefit. However, damage in some joints is the result of unrecognised low-grade infection introduced at the time of the injection. Potent local steroids such as triamcinolone hexacelonide are in use and it must be appreciated that so-called longer-acting steroids are more potent and as such may well be absorbed and cause other problems.

Bier technique

The regional intravenous injection of steroid and local anaesthetic by a method described by Bier for local anaesthetic alone is of use when several joints are affected in one limb (Bier, 1908; Jakubowski, 1973; Salz, 1976).

A double tourniquet with the upper tourniquet inflated is applied below the axilla or around the thigh. Through a butterfly needle a solution of Marcaine is injected intravenously containing 1.5 mg/kg body weight for the arm and 2 mg for the leg or an equivalent dose of Xylocaine. After 2 or 3 minutes the lower cuff is inflated and the upper cuff released. A solution of 50 mg of hydrocortisone for the arm or 100 mg for the leg is injected and the tourniquet kept in position for half an hour. The tourniquet is released intermittently at 5-second intervals to prevent the sudden liberation of a toxic dose of local anaesthetic into the general circulation.

Silicone fluids

These are inert if pure; the oil and grease are excellent lubricants and both have been injected into dry grating rheumatoid joints with a temporary relief of symptoms. Use of the material has,

in the main, been confined to joints destined for surgery to allow the soft tissues to mobilise and to build up muscle power. Many patients seem to experience long-lasting relief of symptoms (Helal and Karadi, 1968). Adverse reaction in the form of a temporary synovitis is exceedingly rare and is probably due to contamination of the material with organic oils.

MODE OF ACTION OF DRUGS IN RELATION TO AETIOLOGY

Drugs used systemically in the treatment of rheumatoid disease are effective in reducing pain and swelling and in some instances reverse serological changes. However, medicines which may to some extent control the manifestations of the disease do not cure it. Moreover their modes of action are not fully understood, for most have several effects of which the comparative significance is unknown.

A knowledge of some of the factors in the pathology of rheumatoid disease helps the surgeon to have at least a working idea of drug action.

Familiarity with aetiological hypotheses of rheumatoid disease will improve communication between physician and surgeon and promote understanding of the mode of action of antirheumatic drugs.

The aetiology of rheumatoid disease is obscure but it is considered that genetic, immunological and/or infective factors take part. The human leucocyte antigen (HLA) system is a series of endogenous antigens found on the surface membranes of human cells. These are genetically determined, the most widely known being HLA B27, which is present in 96 per cent of patients with ankylosing spondylitis and in 11 per cent of the general population (Brewerton, 1976). Work now in progress may show that the D locus HLA antigen is significant in rheumatoid arthritis (Roitt et al., 1978). Infective theories have never been supported by the isolation of a pathogenic organism, perhaps because ribonucleic acid (RNA) of an infecting virus becomes transformed into, and incorporated in, the deoxyribonucleic acid (DNA) of the host cells, where it may remain dormant and unrecognised until activated in suitable conditions.

The numerous drugs which are effective in modifying rheumatoid disease act at various stages in the complex process which culminates in this disease.

The anti-inflammatory agents including gold, deal with the final common path in preventing the release of inflammation-provoking enzymes, and other mediators of inflammation including the prostaglandins. These drugs stabilise the lysosome membrane, preventing its breakdown. Gold salts bind to the plasma proteins, including the immunoglobulin (Ig) complex which forms the rheumatoid factor and penicillamine breaks down the rheumatoid factor into small molecules, both protein-binding and breaking down being mechanisms by which antigenic properties may be destroyed.

The immunosuppressive drugs act by damaging the stem cells of the two lymphocyte families—the B cells, which help confer systemic humoral immunity, and the T cells, which mediate local immunity.

Explanation of the current hypothesis for the pathogenesis of rheumatoid disease starts with the lymphoblast stem cell in the bone marrow (figure 2.2; Roitt *et al.*, 1969).

Some stem cells migrate to the thymus gland and become thymus lymphocytes or T cells. Others remain in the bone marrow, becoming

Figure 2.2 Bone marrow

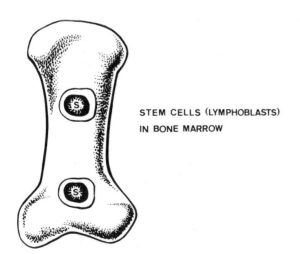

STEM CELLS (LYMPHOBLASTS) IN BONE MARROW

bone marrow lymphocytes, bursal or B cells (figure 2.3).

Bursal cells were so named as their characteristics are similar to those of cells found in the bursa of Fabricius near the egg-laying orifice of chicks (Fabrizzi, 1600). The T and B lymphocytes migrate to the peripheral lymphatic system (figure 2.4).

An antigen enters or becomes attached to these T and B cells, activating them. The origin of this antigen is unknown; it may be exogenous, either bacterial or viral, or it may be endogenous and related to the HLA system (figure 2.5).

The antigen reacts in a complex ill-understood manner with immunoglobulins, which are variously named IgM, IgA, IgG (figure 2.6).

The complexity is such that some of the resulting antibodies themselves act as antigens and a further series of antigen–antibody reactions follow.

The characteristic globulins which appear in some patients with rheumatoid disease are responsible for the serological tests such as Rose Waaler and slide latex.

When an antigen–antibody reaction takes place in the lymphocytes or other sensitised cells, the lysosome membranes are damaged, thus releasing inflammation-producing enzymes. The lysosomes are intracellular bodies arranged around the Golgi apparatus (figure 2.7).

It is these inflammation-producing enzymes which cause the manifestations of rheumatoid disease. The prostaglandins initiate or intensify inflammation; their activity can be estimated and their synthesis or release is inhibited by anti-inflammatory drugs (Saeed *et al.*, 1977; Schneider *et al.*, 1977). Although the lymphocyte has been cited, the polymorphonuclear leucocyte may also play an important part (figure 2.8).

DRUG THERAPY

It is a characteristic of the effective drugs in rheumatoid disease that they have toxic side-effects; and the more effective the drug the more likely it is to be harmful. The toxicity of some drugs makes their exhibition in many patients

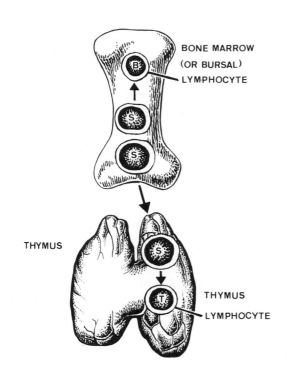

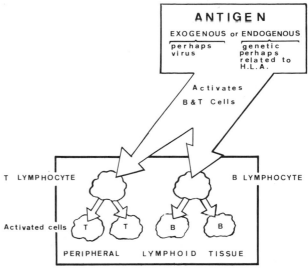

Figure 2.5 The activation of B and T cells by antigen

Figure 2.3 The formation of B and T cells

Figure 2.4 The migration of B and T cells to the peripheral lymphoid tissue

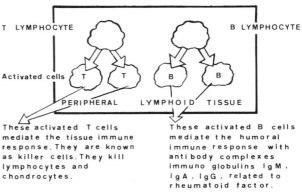

These activated T cells mediate the tissue immune response. They are known as killer cells. They kill lymphocytes and chondrocytes.

These activated B cells mediate the humoral immune response with antibody complexes immuno globulins IgM, IgA, IgG, related to rheumatoid factor.

Figure 2.6 The humoral and tissue immune response

Figure 2.7 Electron microscope structure of the mature lymphocyte to show the lysosomes

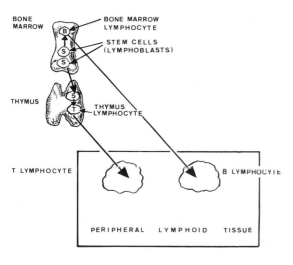

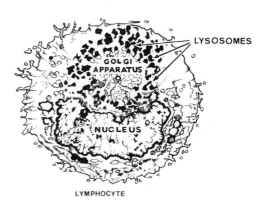

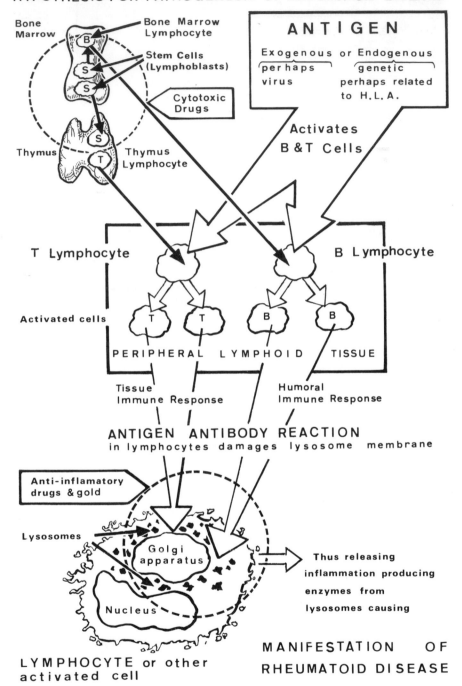

Figure 2.8 Diagram to show the hypothesis for the pathogenesis of rheumatoid disease

totally undesirable, otherwise the treatment can be worse than the disease. The safest drug is given at its lowest effective dose and only when shown to be ineffective at higher doses is another drug tried. Special care is vital for patients with indigestion and peptic ulceration.

Minor non-steroid anti-inflammatory drugs

Minor non-steroid anti-inflammatory drugs such as naproxen, ibuprofen, flurbiprofen are less toxic than aspirin and should be tried first.

Major non-steroid anti-inflammatory drugs

Aspirin is no longer the first choice of anti-rheumatic agents, for when it is given in effective dosage, at least one-third of patients will prove intolerant within 1 month of starting treatment (Mowat, 1977). Aspirin, indomethacin and phenyl-butazone are now considered major non-steroid anti-inflammatory (NSAI) drugs with an import-ant place in later treatment (figure 2.9).

Aspirin stabilises the lysosomal membrane and when given in doses from 650 mg to 1 g four times a day frequently controls the disease, rendering more toxic drugs unnecessary. The side-effects of aspirin may be reduced by enteric-coated prep-arations, by soluble forms of aspirin and by esters such as benorylate. Aspirin should be avoided during pregnancy and in nursing mothers, for it inhibits the blood-clotting mechanism and, owing to the increased possibility of bleeding, it is

Figure 2.9 Flow chart for the drug treatment for rheumatoid disease (from Topics in Therapeutics, *Vol. 3 (Ed. R. G. Shanks), Pitman Medical Publishing Co., Tunbridge Wells, 1976)*

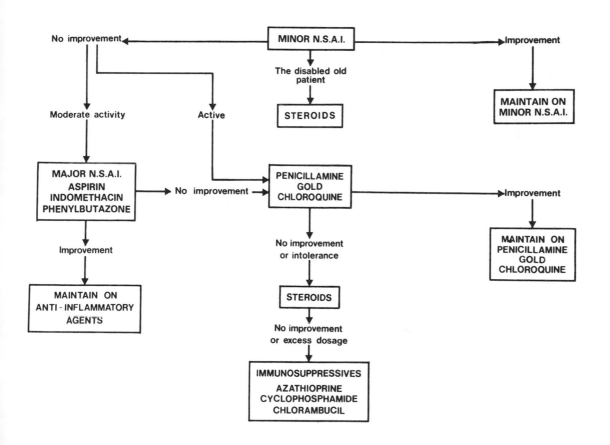

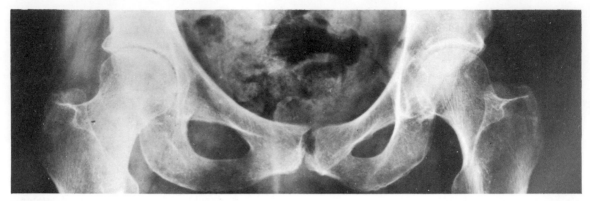

a

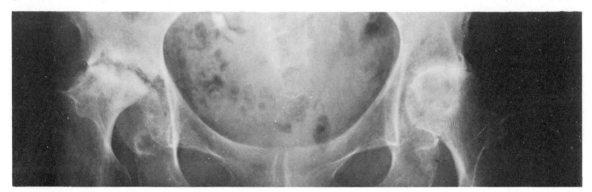

b

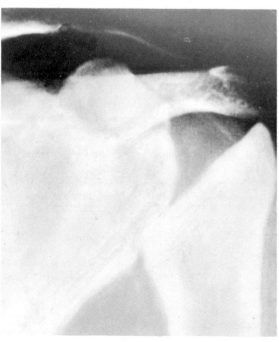

c

Figure 2.10 The Charcot effect of phenylbutazone: (a) and (b), a period of 18 months between these two X-rays; (c) in a shoulder

sometimes stopped 48 hours before operation. On the other hand, some surgeons think that aspirin reduces the incidence of thrombo-embolic complications and prescribe it pre- and post-operatively.

Phenylbutazone decreases capillary permeability and stabilises the lysosome membrane. 100 mg of phenylbutazone is given three times a day for 4 days, and if ineffective, this dose is doubled to 200 mg. After 4 days, if still ineffective, the drug is stopped, but if effective, the dose is reduced. This principle of administering medicines is applied to many of the anti-inflammatory drugs, which are only continued if therapeutically effective. A close watch is kept on the blood for dyscrasias.

Indomethacin inhibits both leucocyte and polymorph activity. It is particularly useful in reducing morning stiffness with a dose of 50–100 mg at night.

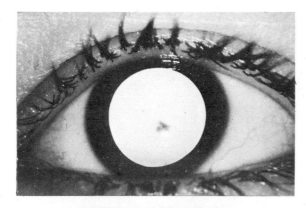

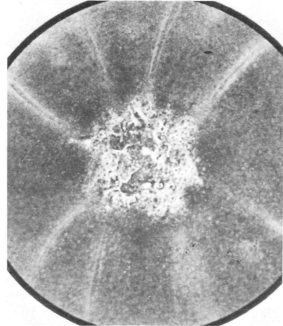

Figure 2.11 Posterior capsular cataract occurring in a patient on long–term steroid therapy (B. Ansell and The Institute of Ophthalmology)

Both phenylbutazone and indomethacin are irritant to the gastric mucosa and must be exhibited with caution in patients with a history of peptic ulcer. When prescribed orally, they should always be taken with meals, not before or after. When the stomach is unduly affected by phenylbutazone and indomethacin, these drugs may be given in the form of suppositories. In this form they are less likely to irritate the gastric mucosa, but care is still necessary, as fatal gastric haemorrhage has followed the rectal administration of these drugs.

The analgesic properties of these drugs are sometimes so powerful that rapid changes occur similar to those seen in Charcot joints. The appearances are characteristic (figure 2.10) and are due to the effectiveness of the anti-inflammatory agent in suppressing protective pain (Sweetnam, Mason and Murray, 1960; Murray and Jacobson, 1972).

Gold salts

Gold stabilises the lysosomal membrane by binding to the plasma proteins, including the rheumatoid factor, and will sometimes convert a sero-positive case to sero-negative. In small doses toxic effects are less common, and if there are no adverse reactions, gold may be given indefinitely. The onset of a skin rash is the signal to stop the drug, although it may be tried again later.

Corticosteroids

Long-term systemic corticosteroids should be avoided in rheumatoid disease whenever possible. These drugs have no beneficial effects on the

TABLE 2.1 UNWANTED EFFECTS OF CORTICOSTEROIDS

These include
  Acute pancreatitis
  Peptic ulcer
  Osteoporosis
  Diabetes
  Hypertension (particularly from ACTH)
  Liability to infection
  Reactivation of quiescent tuberculosis
  Posterior capsular cataract
  Adrenocortical atrophy and loss of response to
    stress with possible hypotensive crisis
  Vascular lesions, increased fragility, polyarteritis
  Connective tissue and skin friability
  Muscle atrophy
  Steroid acne
  Moon facies
  Dowager's hump
  Supraclavicular pads
  Other deposition of fat
  Overweight
  Fluid retention
  Facial erythema
  Psychiatric disturbances
  Vaccination complications

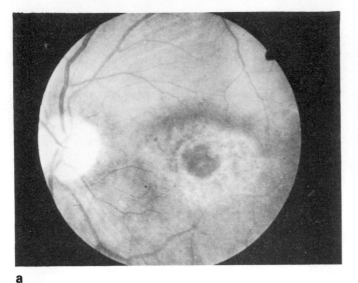

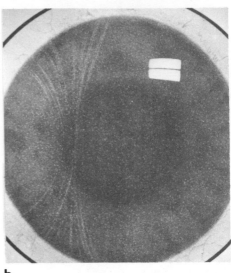

a   **b**

Figure 2.12 (a) A bull's eye fundus due to retinal pigmentation in a patient on chloroquine (B. Ansell); (b) a chloroquine cornea (The Institute of Ophthalmology)

ultimate course of the disease, and not only have serious toxic effects, but also compound the ill-effects of the disease in weakening skin and connective tissue, including bones (table 2.1; figure 2.11). Systemic corticosteroids also increase the morbidity following surgery. If long-term corticosteroids are necessary, every effort should be made to keep the daily dose down to 5 mg. In the event of an injury, an operation or an acute illness unrelated to rheumatoid disease, the patient on long-term corticosteroids may develop an acute Addisonian hypotensive crisis. During such a period of risk supplemental corticosteroid may be given. Short courses of systemic corticosteroids appear to be harmless; they are sometimes effective in otherwise intractable neck pain and corticosteroids are the treatment of choice in poly-myalgia rheumatica. Temporal arteritis is an acute medical emergency and when diagnosed the consequent hazard of blindness may be averted by corticosteroids.

ACTH

Adrenocorticotropic hormone acts by stimulating the production of corticosteroids and presents

similar dangers to those of prolonged corticosteroid administration except that the adrenal cortex does not atrophy (table 2.1).

Chloroquine

This antimalarial drug stabilises the lysosomal membrane and in the long term may reverse serological changes. However, it can induce serious optical effects; the corneal changes (figure 2.12b) are reversible but the retinal changes may be permanent. The drug is deposited in the macula and is associated with retinal pigmentation, giving the characteristic retinoscopic appearance of a bull's eye (figure 2.12a). Hydrochloroquine has replaced chloroquine but is not free from eye complications, for blindness occurs in 1 in 1000–2000 cases. The risk may be acceptable when balanced against the risks of other drugs (Marks and Power, 1979). Three-monthly examinations by an ophthalmic surgeon are mandatory.

Penicillamine

This breaks down the large rheumatoid factor molecule and positive serology may be reversed; surprisingly its beneficial effect may not be due to this mechanism. Penicillamine has numerous toxic effects affecting one-third of all patients treated. It is too early to assess its role but it is effective sometimes in severe rheumatoid disease with vasculitis. When prescribed, the blood and urine need continuous monitoring.

Immuno-suppressive agents

Cyclophosphamide, a nitrogen mustard, and methotrexate, a folic acid antagonist, act by interfering with the metabolism of rapidly dividing cells. They are radiomimetic and damage the lymphoblast ' precursors of the T and B lymphocytes.

These drugs take 6 weeks to initiate clinical benefit and improvement continues for 3–4 months; the toxicity is considerable, and immunosuppressive agents are only used when less risky methods fail, for all rapidly growing cells may be damaged and the entire haemopoietic system put at risk. Nausea and alopecia may occur. Chromosome analysis reveals an increase in abnormalities from 4.6 to 13.8 per cent but this returns to normal after discontinuing the drug. However, long-term serious possibilities such as infertility and teratogenesis must be borne in mind.

REFERENCES

Bier, A. (1908). *Arch. Klin. Chir.*, **86,** 1007

Brewerton, D. A. (1976). HLA B27 and the inheritance of susceptibility to rheumatic disease. *Arth. Rheum.*, **19**(5), 656

Fabrizzi Girolamo (Fabricius ab Aquapendente) (1600). *De formation foetu*, Venetiis per F. Bolzettam

Helal, B. and Karadi, B. S. (1968). Artificial lubrication of joints. *Ann. Phys. Med.*, **IX**(8), 334–340

Jakubowski, S. (1973). The use of Bier's technique for regional hydrocortisone. Personal communication

Maitland, G. D. (1970). *Peripheral Manipulation*, Butterworths, London

Marks, J. S. and Power, B. J. (1979). Is chloroquine obsolete in treatment of rheumatoid disease. Lancet, **i,** 371–373

Mennell, J. B. (1960). *Physical Treatment by Movement, Manipulation and Massage*, 5th edn, Churchill, London

Mowat, A. G. (1977). Rational approach to the use of non-steroid anti-inflammatory drugs. *Topics in Therapeutics*, Vol. 3 (ed. Shanks, R. G.), Pitman Medical, London, pp. 76–86

Murray, R. O. and Jacobson, H. G. (1972). *The Radiology of Skeletal Disorders*, Churchill Livingston, Edinburgh, p. 658

Roitt, I. M., Greaves, M. F., Torrigiani, G. Brostoff, J. and Playfair, J. H. L. (1969). The cellular basis of immunological responses. *Lancet*, August 16, 367

Roitt, I. M., Corbett, M., Festenstein, H., Jaraquemada, D., Papasteriadis, C., Hay, F. C. and Nineam, L. J. (1978). HLA-DRW4 and prognosis in rheumatoid arthritis. *Lancet*, 6 May, 990

Saeed, S. A., McDonald-Gibson, W. J., Cuthbert, J., Copas, J. L., Schneider, C., Gardiner, P. J., Butt, N. M. and Collier, H.O.J. (1977). Endogenous inhibitor of prostaglandin synthetase. *Nature*, **270,** 32–36

Salz, M. (1976). Bier's technique for regional hydrocortisone. Mtg *Rheum. Arth. Surg. Soc.*, Toronto October

Swanson, N. (1977). *Bull. Orth. Arth. Hosp.*, *Toronto*, **X**(1), 4

Sweetnam, D. R., Mason, R. M. and Murray, R. O. (1960). Steroid arthropathy of the hip. *Br. Med. J.* **1,** 1392

3

PERIOPERATIVE CARE

A surgical procedure is but an incident in the overall care of the patient. Improvement of one aspect to the detriment of the whole is unacceptable; hence the great importance of assessment and judgement.

Pre-operative assessment and investigation must be thorough and comprehensive, for it is only when the patient's particular problems have been defined that the best solution can be calculated and errors of judgement avoided.

Impressions are not only unreliable, but are also positively misleading, and memory is fickle. It is, therefore, important to record both subjective and objective findings. Photography and the tape recorder are useful adjuncts to the clinical account.

HISTORY-TAKING

This should be systematically taken, starting with the patient's present complaint. The story of the disease from its onset will guide the investigator as to severity and prognosis; for example, the duration of morning stiffness, pain assessed in terms of the analgesic requirements and, most impor-

tant, the drug treatment with especial reference to steroids, since a patient on systemic steroid therapy may require extra steroid cover for any operation contemplated.

Specific enquiry must always be made regarding the state of the neck in anticipation of an anaesthetic. In a polysystemic disease, enquiry into the general state of health with specific reference to each system is important.

The history is elicited by specific questioning as to previous serious illness, accidents or operations.

The social history should seek information about habits, economic and domestic problems, including the subject's sexual activity. The degree of independence and ability to carry out work and hobbies is all-important in deciding upon a line of treatment. The family history must be recorded, including details of the support the patient is likely to obtain at home.

EXAMINATION

This must be thorough and encompass all systems. It must be remembered that synovial joints are

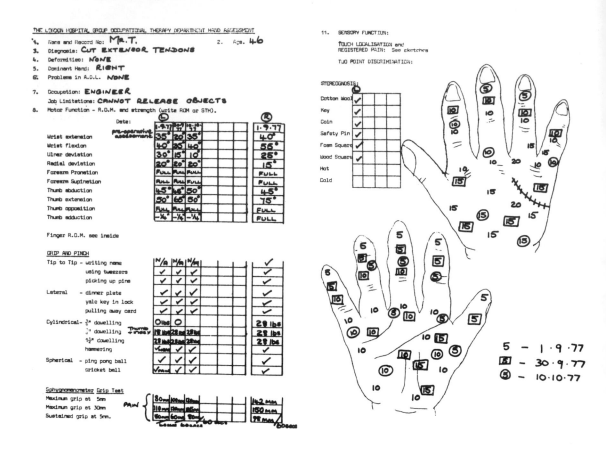

Figure 3.1 Hand assessment charts. These tests are carried out by the occupational therapists

involved in the process of phonation (crico-arytenoid) and hearing (interossicular). The rheumatoid nodule and the arteritic lesion can affect numerous structures, as can the complication of amyloidosis.

A psychological assessment and judgement of the degree of motivation is important. There should be no hesitancy in seeking expertise. Psychologists, social workers (who can assess the patients in their home environment) rheumatologists, ophthalmic surgeons, chest physicians, haematologists, immunologists and many other specialists frequently assist in the overall management of the patient.

THE LOCOMOTOR STATE

A review of fixed deformity, of the measurement of power and of the range of movement is valuable, but more important is the ability to carry out the function required of the part. For example, arthrodesis of the wrist may produce little disability though all movement is lost.

Power is assessed quantitatively by performance of an action against a known resistance. Movements can be measured by compass or protractor or by the distance from a fixed point that can be reached—for example, heel to buttock in limited knee flexion. The range of movement can be accurately traced in the finger by the use of Odstock wire tracings. In these, malleable wire is bent over the finger in full flexion and extension and the shape taken traced on to paper. A different colour is used for each subsequent measurement,

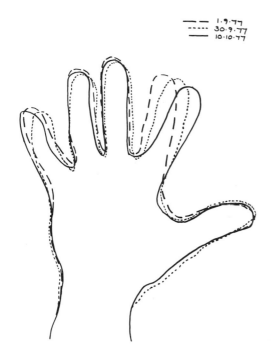

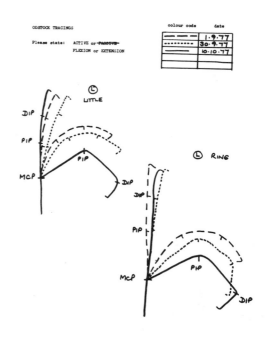

together with dates of measurement. This provides an accurate pictorial progress (figure 3.1). A 'cosmetic' assessment should also be made in trying to determine a surgical approach or type of prosthesis.

It is useful to have mock-ups of home within the hospital (figure 3.2) so that the ability to stand, walk, sit, wash, dress, cook, feed and use crutches can be assessed by a suitably trained worker, such as an occupational therapist or social worker.

ASSESSMENT OF THE GENERAL ACTIVITY OF THE DISEASE

Inflammatory state

Factors to be considered are

(1) Morning Stiffness.
(2) Grip strength.
(3) Number of active joints.
(4) Erythrocyte sedimentation rate.
(5) Thermography.

The severity of the disease

The damage/duration index. For example:

10 damaged joints; 5 years disease duration = 10/5 = 2

10 damaged joints; 40 years disease duration = 10/40 = 0.25

An average value is 0.75.

The severity of joint damage

b/X-ray indices 1–6 (Larsen, 1973).
These range from normal to total joint destruction and require X-ray templates for joints commonly involved, with which it is easy to match the patient's films (figure 3.3).

SPECIAL INVESTIGATIONS

Blood tests. Haemoglobin, white cell count, sedimentation rate or plasma viscosity and latex are the basic tests. It is sensible if surgery is

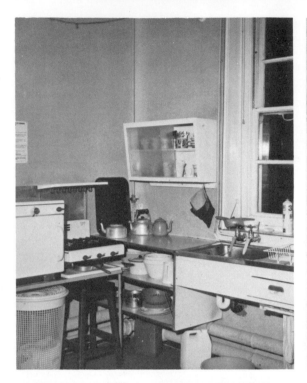
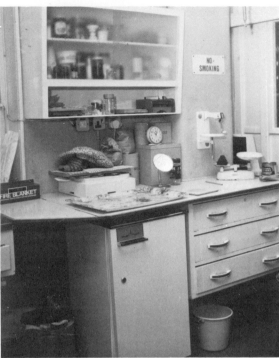
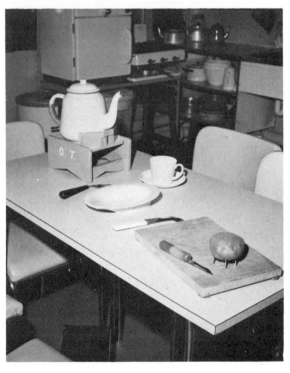
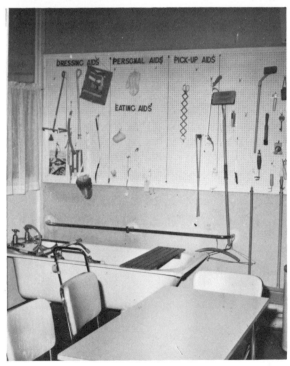

Figure 3.2 Mock-up of home and aids to daily living (Occupational Therapy, Highlands Hospital)

SHOULDER

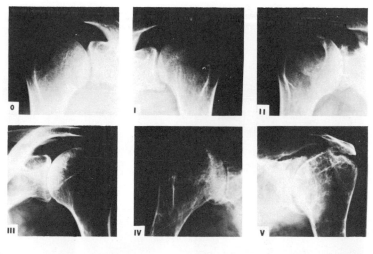

ELBOW

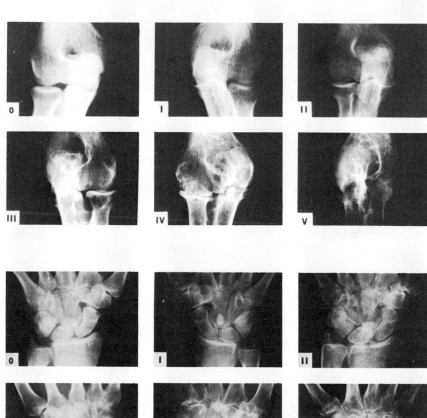

WRIST

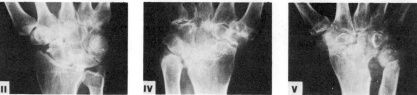

Figure 3.3 Standard series of grades of joint damage (A. Larsen)

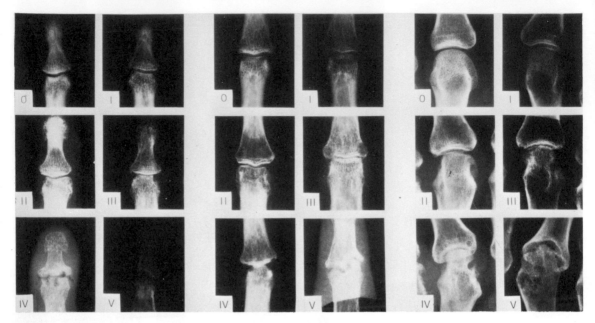

FINGERS

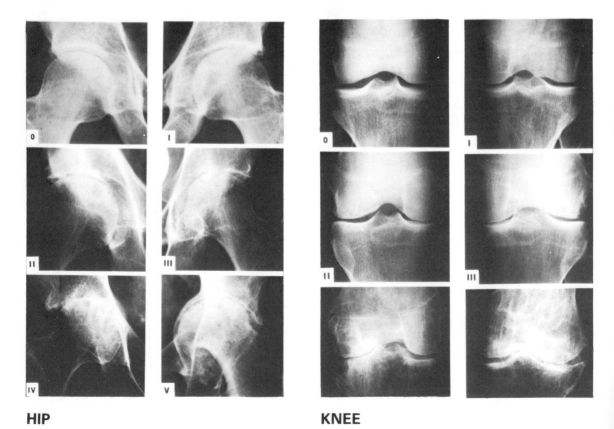

HIP   **KNEE**

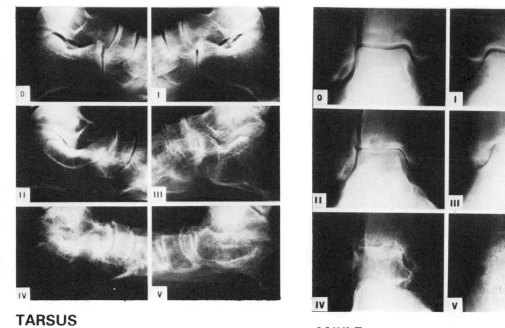

TARSUS

ANKLE

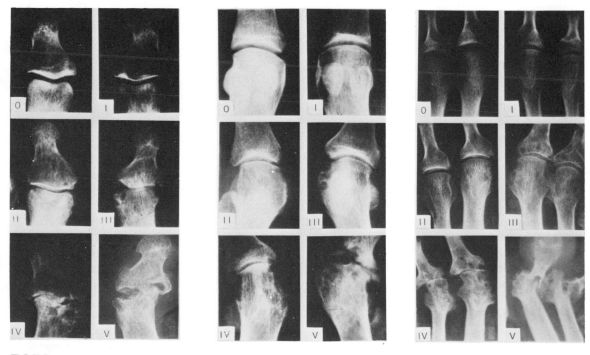

TOES

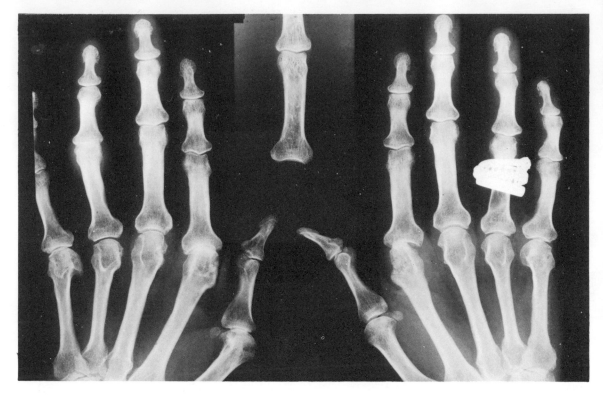

Figure 3.4 Cadaver finger for standard porosity comparison

contemplated to ask for the patient to be grouped at the same time. In spondylitis, tests such as the human leucocyte antigen B27 (HLA B27) can support the diagnosis.

X-rays of the affected part and a routine chest X-ray are taken. X-rays of hands and spine against a standard porosity are sometimes of help in assessing osteoporosis (figure 3.4).

Tomography will reveal hidden subarticular cysts. Contrast media may be necessary in the spine and in arthrograms of the shoulder, knee or other joints. Cineradiography may be of great value after contrast injection.

Technetium scanning can be useful in identifying specific portions of a joint that are affected (figure 3.5; Plate 1) or inflammation around one component of a prosthesis.

EMI scan (Computerised axial tomography). Although not in general use, as yet, the detail possible is impressive. It is particularly useful in spinal work and in identifying bone damage. The technique will eventually replace tomography (figure 3.6).

Cineradiography, particularly in association with myelography, is extremely useful in identifying spinal instability and root impingement.

Thermography (Ring *et al.*, 1974). Temperatures can be measured to within 2°C by a thermograph; this will accurately outline, for example, areas of synovitis within a particular joint and is an index of the efficiency of treatment (figure 3.7; Plate 2).

Gait analysis requires a walkway connected to a recording device; it provides a good comparative measure of progress but is at present mainly an experimental device.

Arthroscopy. The arthroscope allows a direct view of the interior of joints. This can be carried out on quite small joints such as the metacarpophalangeal joint if a needle arthroscope is used.

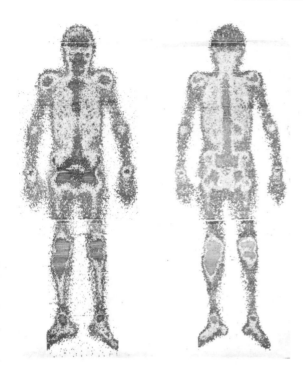

Figure 3.5 Whole-body technetium scan showing multiple joint inflammation (R. Wighton). See plate I

Commonly it is used in the knee and shoulder and can be used to biopsy synovial membrane (Helal and Chen, 1976).

Photography. Moving film and videotaping can provide an excellent record.

ASSESSMENT OF PRIORITIES

In a multi-system and multi-joint disease it is of great importance to plan the management to the patient's best advantage. Priorities are determined by life-endangering situations: for example, an unstable neck, which may at any time produce death or tetraplegia, should be dealt with first. If lower limb surgery is necessary and crutches have to be used, then the state of the upper limb joints should be remedied first. Situations which will result in further damage to tissues and, if neglected, will demand more complex surgery have the next highest priority: for example, dorsal extensor

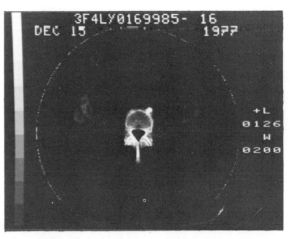

Figure 3.6 EMI scan outlining spinal facetal joints (L. Kreel)

synovitis or a caput ulnae syndrome or a flexor tenosynovitis with potential or impending tendon rupture. Finally, in deciding between hip, knee and ankle or foot surgery the proximal joints usually take precedence as alignment of one affects the other. An adducted hip can rapidly ruin a knee prosthesis by subjecting it to intolerable valgus strain (figure 13.17).

THE IMMEDIATE PRE-OPERATIVE PERIOD

The immediate pre-operative period is perhaps the most stressful time for a patient. Encouragement, explanation and relieving fear of pain will produce rewards in patient co-operation. Familiarisation with exercises which will be necessary immediately post-operatively is essential, particularly breathing exercises, anti-thrombotic exercises and exercises specifically chosen to rehabilitate the part or the patient as a whole. Patients with potential instability of the neck should be placed in a collar support if only to alert the anaesthetist. The part to be operated upon is indelibly marked. Steroid supplements are charted and given when necessary. An antibiotic, if advised, is commenced and given with the premedication. Elasticated stockings are put on to keep the calf veins empty and prevent thrombosis.

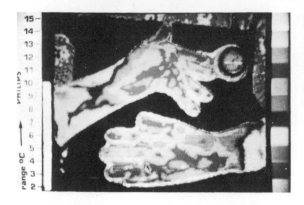

Figure 3.7 Thermogram showing rheumatoid disease of 10 years' duration. Proximal interphalangeal joints of right index (upper hand) and left 4th and 5th fingers are inflamed (E.F.J. Ring and H.A. Bird). See plate 2

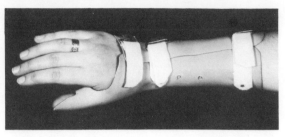

Figure 3.8 Rigid resting splint for wrist and thumb (M. Ellis, Tower Hamlets District Occupational Therapist)

CARE DURING SURGERY

(1) Gentle tissue handling is important in a collagen disease where there is fragility which may have been further aggravated by steroids. Under anaesthaesia passive movements which would not affect normal bones may result in fractures in the rheumatoid subject.

(2) (a) The arrest of haemorrhage and haematoma prevention by meticulous haemostasis is the next priority. Small vessels near the skin are best treated by a bipolar coagulator which is more local in its action than diathermy and so causes less tissue damage. (b) Vacuum drainage. (c) Careful pressure bandaging. (d) Elevation. (e) Careful suturing of the skin. The outcome of a well-executed surgical procedure can be ruined by the terrible triad of haematoma, wound dehiscence or skin necrosis and infection. This calamity is especially disastrous following implant surgery.

(3) The integrity of the circulation is ensured by careful bandaging and splinting, yet there should be adequate exposure of the hands and feet for the inspection of skin circulation.

(4) There should be a fine balance between the use of analgesics and soporifics—that is between comfort and overdosage. Respiratory depression must be avoided, as must prolonged immobility. The patient's level of consciousness should be such as to allow full sensible co-operation.

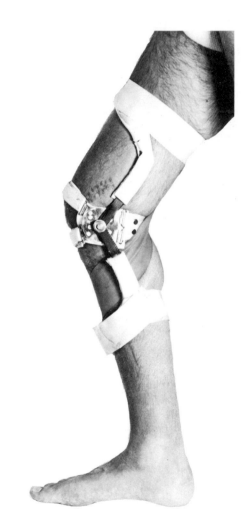

Figure 3.9 Mobile splint to protect against collateral and rotational movement (M. Ellis, Tower Hamlets District Occupational Therapist)

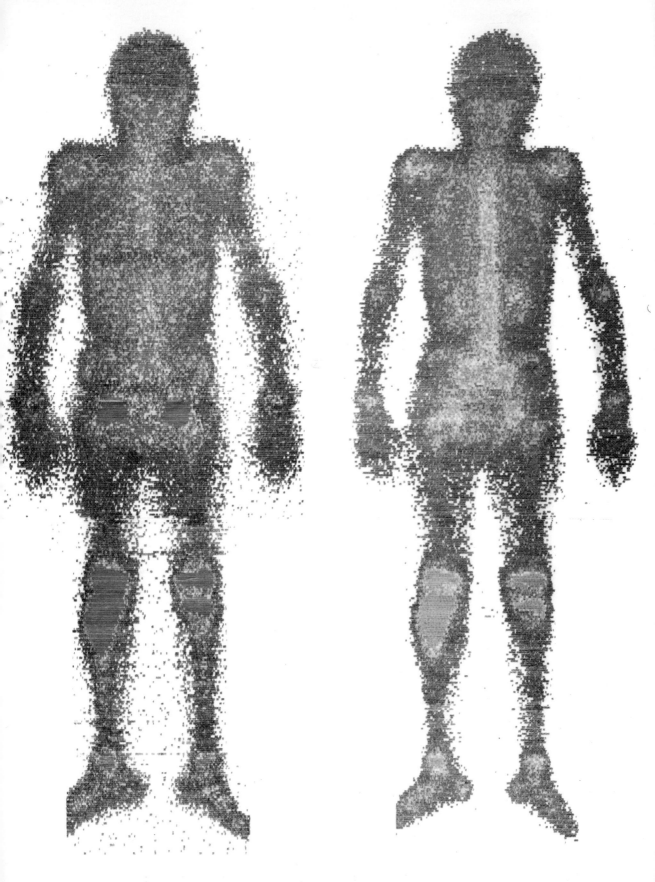

Plate 1. Whole-body technetium scan showing multiple joint inflammation. Left, anterior view; right, posterior view (R. Wighton)

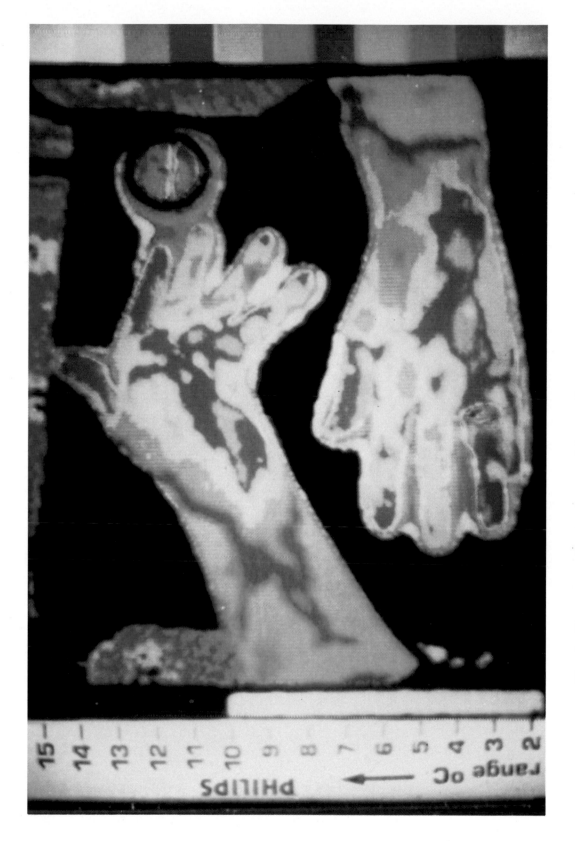

Plate 2. Thermogram showing rheumatoid disease of 10 years' duration. Proximal interphalangeal joints of right index (upper hand) and left 4th and 5th fingers are inflamed (E.F.J. Ring and H.A. Bird)

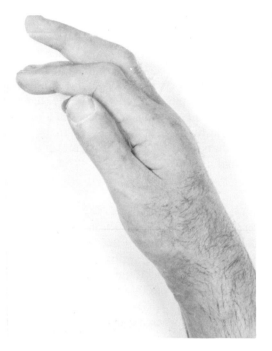

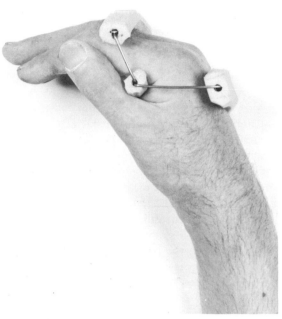

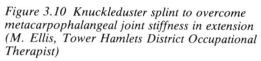

Figure 3.10 Knuckleduster splint to overcome metacarpophalangeal joint stiffness in extension (M. Ellis, Tower Hamlets District Occupational Therapist)

(5) Post-operative swelling must be minimised by careful pressure bandaging, elevation and exercise. The proper control of steroids and attention to anaemia, plasma proteins and electrolyte balance will eliminate oedema from these sources.

(6) The incidence of post-operative venous thrombosis may be reduced by care to avoid undue compression to limbs during surgery. Thrombosis is diminished by elasticated support or more sophisticated means such as calf pump, salicylates, Vitamin C, other anticoagulants and early mobilisation. Early recognition of thrombosis, if it occurs, is essential and is best recognised by a rise in skin temperature of the affected limb, for systemic temperature rise, calf pain and oedema are relatively late.

(7) Deformity, or damage to the surgical repair or reconstruction is avoided by careful splintage which may be either static or mobile and is designed to avoid contractures.

POST-OPERATIVE CARE

(1) Relief of tension on the skin until this is properly healed is essential, the part being immobilised if necessary.

(2) Remobilisation of all joints that can be moved is started immediately. A graduated programme of exercises aided by occupational therapy is ideal.

(3) The patient's stay in the hospital environment should be as short as is practicable. Home circumstances must be surveyed and if necessary supplemented by home help, visits from the district nurse, etc. Facilities such as lavatories on each floor are assessed, and cleaning and cooking and sleeping problems are defined with a view to providing aids to daily living.

(4) Assessment for a return to work is made with the help of occupational therapists and social workers. Retraining programmes can be arranged.

(5) Supervision of the general rheumatoid state, medication, etc., and of the progress of the patient, with special reference to the surgery, is carried out. This follow-up is best conducted in the combined clinic, at which the patient can have a simultaneous contact with his rheumatologist and surgeon.

(6) Splints may be an essential adjuvant to the treatment at any stage and indispensable for a period especially post-operatively. External splints are basically of three types, which are (a) rigid (figure 3.8); (b) allow movements at the joints (figure 3.9); (c) allow movements at the joints and exert force (figure 3.10).

Many materials are used in splint construction, and among the factors to be considered are weight, strength, compatibility with the skin in that they must be non-irritant, cost and the ease with which the material can be worked. Generally, splints should be made to measure (Mannerfelt and Fredriksson, 1976). Many ingenious methods have been devised: inflatable splints and splints made of particulate material in an enclosed system are moulded to the part to be splinted and then made rigid by creating a vacuum which bonds the particles firmly together. An important consideration is the patient's ability to apply and remove the splint, and in this connection the Velcro fastening has proved a boon.

Splints are needed for the following reasons:

(1) *To discourage movement.* (a) Limitation of abnormal movement: In a long bone after a fracture, or in a joint following ligamentous or bony damage. Joint instability is commonly encountered in rheumatoid arthritis after synovial distension or synovial destruction of the ligaments or subchondral bone. Splints are also applied to prevent deformity due to everyday stresses; a typical example of a working splint is the rigid elbow support (figure 3.11). (b) Limitation of normal joint movement: Rigid splints can be used simply to rest inflamed joints and relieve pain, or to prevent inflamed joints from developing contractures by splinting in a position which will allow the limb as a whole to function optimally, or alternatively in a position where the capsule and ligaments are kept out to length. Finally, such splintage may be used to stabilise one or more joints in a linked system of joints to permit movement and power in one joint which is left free of restriction (figure 3.12).

(2) *To encourage movement while providing support for joints or bones.* In a polyarthritis it is generally desirable to keep joints mobile in order to avoid stiffness, which will in its turn throw inordinate stress on those joints that remain functional. Splints prevent deformity (figure 3.13) as well as adventitious movement in a joint made unstable by juxta-articular bony or by ligamentous damage, while permitting movement in the normal arc.

(3) *To assist movement.* These splints provide dynamic force in the direction required either by the intrinsic elasticity of the material (figure 3.14) or by incorporating spring wire (figure 3.15) or elastic into the splint (figure 3.16). They are used to assist weak or paralysed muscles, to overcome fixed deformity, or to protect a repair, on the principle that when a muscle contracts, its antagonist actively relaxes. This is particularly useful in maintaining joint movement while protecting a tendon repair.

(4) *To simulate a post-operative state.* To give patients an idea as to what they can manage after an operation such as an arthrodesis, a rigid splint can be applied, commonly to the knee, wrist or ankle. It will also from time to time allow an assessment of the clinical response—for example, pain relief. Pre-operative dynamic bracing can also give some guide as to the effect of, for example, an anticipated tendon transposition operation.

FORMS

Forms such as that outlined on pages 36–37 and that shown in figure 3.1 are a useful aid to memory and can be valuable in retrospective research.

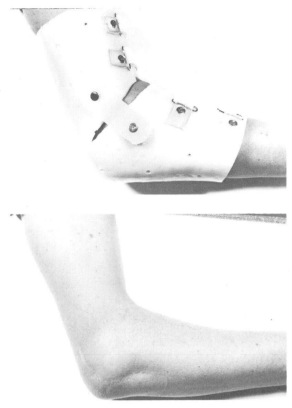

Figure 3.11 Elbow working splint (M. Ellis, Tower Hamlets District Occupational Therapist)

Figure 3.13 Splint to prevent ulnar drift (M. Ellis, Tower Hamlets District Occupational Therapist)

Figure 3.12 Splint to stabilise wrist and metacarpophalangeal joints in order to allow power and movement to be concentrated on the interphalangeal joints (M. Ellis, Tower Hamlets District Occupational Therapist)

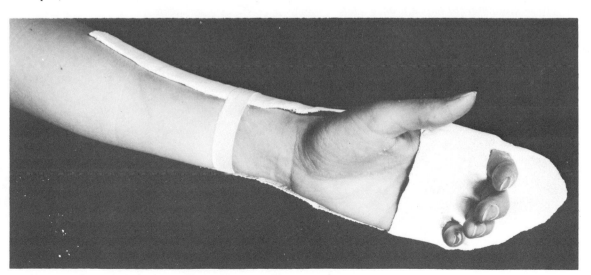

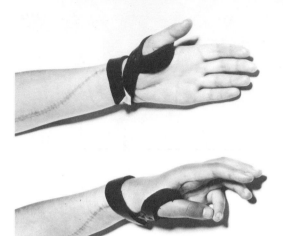

Figure 3.14 Rubber splint to aid opposition of thumb (M. Ellis, Tower Hamlets District Occupational Therapist)

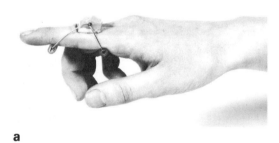

a

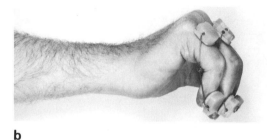

b

Figure 3.15 Splints incorporating wire springs (M. Ellis, Tower Hamlets District Occupational Therapist): (a) Odstock splint to extend proximal interphalangeal joint; (b) to flex proximal interphalangeal joints; (c) wrist drop spring splint

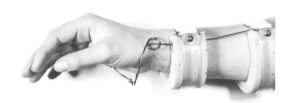

c

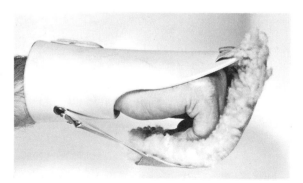

Figure 3.16 Flexor cuff (M. Ellis, Tower Hamlets District Occupational Therapist)

A form for recording general information

Name	Sex	Date of birth	Age	
Address		Family doctor		Examiner
Occupation		Hobbies		

		Juvenile	
Diagnosis	Rheumatoid		Osteo, psoriatic, ankylosing, other
		Adult	

Family history		Work records, times off	length	
		sudden		peripheral
Date of onset	Mode		Distribution	central
		gradual		both
Blood tests	Hb.	WBC	ESR	Latex	HLA B27

X-rays – tomography	Photographs	Films
contrast media	prints	8mm
cineradiography	slides	16mm
thermography		
isotopes, eg. technetium scan		
EMI scan		
gait analyser		
arthroscopy		

Local locomotor assessment – pain	Joints involved
warmth	man diagram
swelling	
crepitus	
movements	
stability	
alignment	
power	

Disease severity – damage/duration index X-ray grading
Inflammatory state – morning stiffness
    grip strength
    number of active joints

Treatments	Systemic	salicylates	
		phenylbutazone	
		indomethacin	
		gold	
		antimalarial	
		immunosuppressive	
		steroids	
	Local	intra-articular injections:	anti-inflammatory
			chemical
			radioactive colloid
			lubricant
		splintage	
		operation	
	Bed rest	hospital	
		home	
Operation site	Joint	synovectomy	
		arthroplasty	
		osteotomy	
		arthrodesis	
		tenodesis	
		dermodesis	
		capsulorrhaphy	*(continued on p. 38)*

Tendon

synovectomy
repair
release
transfer
tenodesis
graft

Other

Post-operative complications

local

infection
haematoma
dehiscence
adhesion .
necrosis

systemic

neurological
cardiovascular
respiratory
genito-urinary
alimentary
peripheral circulatory
locomotor

Functional assessment
  Sleep   in and out of bed
  Toilet
  Groom   wash and bath – teeth
                         hair
                         shave
                         cut nails
  Dressing
Walk – alone
       assisted
       wheelchair
       bed
       shop
       public transport
       stairs
       work: housework, cooking, driving
Leisure activity – hobby
                   sport

Post-operative assessment

REFERENCES

Helal, B. and Chen, S. C. (1976). Arthroscopy of the knee, *Br. J. Hosp. Med.*, June, 583–595

Larsen, A. (1973). Radiological grading of rheumatoid arthritis, an observer study. *Scand. J. Rheum.*, **2,** 136

Larsen, A., Dale, K. and Eek, M. (1977). Radiographic evaluation of rheumatoid arthritis and related conditions by standard reference forms. *Acta Radiol. Diagnosis*, 481–491

Mannerfelt, L. and Fredriksson, K. (1976). The effect of commercial orthoses on rheumatically deformed hands, *S.T.U. Report*, No. 47

Ring, E. E. L., Collins, A. J., Bacon, P. A. and Cosh, J. A. (1974). Quantitation of thermography in arthritis using multi-isothermal analysis. *Ann. Rheum. Dis.*, **33,** 353–356

4

SYNOVECTOMY

No procedure has given rise to more controversy than synovectomy. In the natural history of rheumatoid arthritis there is fluctuation in disease activity: further modification results from emotional and environmental factors and from systemic medical and physical treatments; thus a valid scientific assessment of the outcome of synovectomy is virtually impossible. The consensus of opinion, however, is that synovectomy results in improvement of local disease activity and so delays deterioration (Report ARC and BOA, 1976).

DAMAGE PRODUCED BY SYNOVITIS

In joints

In the joints, hypertrophy produces distension, so stretching the capsuloligamentous complex, and on subsiding, leaves instability. The synovium undermines the subarticular bone and results in erosions and weakness which may cause fracture, collapse and further instability and deformity. It may by intrusion between articular surfaces in-terfere with the nutrition of the cartilage and also obstruct joint movement. It produces lysosomes which form cathepsins capable of destroying articular cartilage. Synovitis of a joint may occasionally result in nerve compression when nerves traverse a confined space adjacent to the joint. Classical examples are the ulnar nerve in its passage behind the medial epicondyle of the humerus and the posterior interosseous nerve as it skirts the radial head.

Around tendons

At this site the problems are twofold. Firstly, synovitis may produce a direct effect on the tendon by compression where the tendon passes into the confines of a retinaculum or sheath; this may eventually cause rupture by pressure necrosis (figure 4.1). Sites at which this occurs are the dorsal extensor compartment of the wrist, the mouths of the flexor sheaths (figure 4.2) and the carpal tunnel. Secondly, other structures sharing passage with the tendon in a confined space can be compressed, the most vulnerable generally being a nerve. A common site is in the carpal tunnel at the

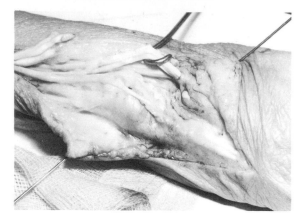

Figure 4.1 Compression rupture of tendons in the extensor compartment of the wrist due to synovitis

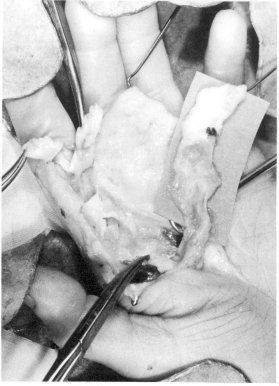

Figure 4.2 Rupture of flexor tendon at the mouth of the fibrous flexor sheath

wrist, where the median nerve is compressed; another is the tarsal tunnel behind the medial malleolus, where the posterior tibial nerve may be entrapped.

In bursae

Here the effects are usually due to direct pressure causing discomfort. This is common over bony points such as the olecranon (figure 4.3), the greater trochanter, the patella and the Achilles tendon insertion. Bursae which connect with joints, such as popliteal bursae, will only settle after synovectomy of the joint itself, and it must be emphasised that simple excision of the bursa never suffices in such a situation (figure 14.10, p. 179).

Epiphyses

Synovitis, because of the greatly increased blood flow resulting from the inflammatory response, can produce overgrowth of bone in the child. Occasionally uneven growth causes malalignments (figure 4.5).

Systemic

The synovium may be the site of antigen formation in rheumatoid disease and it is not uncommon to obtain a general systemic remission of the disease after removal of a substantial bulk of synovium.

TREATMENTS OF SYNOVITIS AND SYNOVIAL HYPERTROPHY

(1) Anti-inflammatory medicines given systemically or locally into the joint.

(2) Simple external physical means—cooling, rest or splintage.

(3) Chemical agents introduced locally to produce destruction of the synovium.

(4) Physical agents introduced locally to destroy the synovium.

(5) By indirectly reducing the blood supply, as in double osteotomy at the knee.

(6) Surgical excision of the synovium.

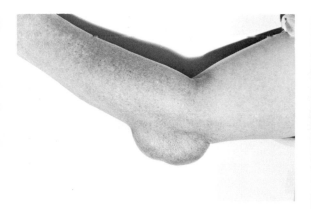

Figure 4.3 Olecranon bursa

Many treatments have long-term deleterious effects which may still appear in the future. Apart from surgery, the methods which aim to reduce inflammation and those which produce destruction of synovium are unfortunately not highly tissue-selective and may also damage articular cartilage. The systemic effects of radiation and radioactive materials can be hazardous in the long term.

Synovial ablation

There is some measure of agreement that surgical and non-surgical synovectomy should be contemplated only when adequate medical treatment, including systemic anti-inflammatory medicines and simple physical measures such as rest, cooling or splintage, have been tried for at least 3–4 months without response. It should be noted, however, that local steroid treatment has been shown by Salter and Murray (1969) to produce articular cartilage damage in animals, and remote and local complications have been reported, such as cutaneous atrophy (Cassidy and Boyle, 1966). Some caution is advised, particularly against too frequent injections. Three injections at 3-week intervals in any 6-month period is the maximum we allow.

In children non-surgical synovectomy carries with it important risks. Surgical synovectomy should not be performed under the age of 6, principally because of severe joint stiffness which ensues, unless there is good patient co-operation in

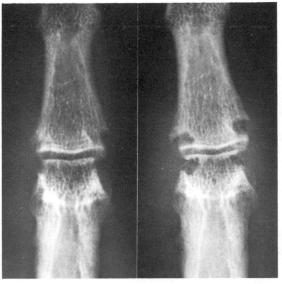

a   b

Figure 4.4 X-rays of proximal interphalangeal joint immediately before (a) and immediately after (b) synovectomy. Debris-filled cavities have become obvious after surgical synovectomy

rehabilitation. Each child should be separately assessed, for a particularly well-motivated and co-operative child can be treated at an earlier age. Although it is generally stated that joints with erosive changes are not suitable for synovectomy, this has not been our experience provided there is a good range of movement and only moderate instability. It should be noted that in many assessments an immediate post-operative X-ray has not been taken and thus disease progression may be falsely reported. Many early erosions still contain bone debris and synovium which masks the erosive cavity in the immediate pre-operative X-ray. Upon removal of synovium within the cavity together with bone debris, the cavity becomes evident on X-ray; this, we feel, is one of the factors which produce case reports of deterioration when X-rays are taken months later and therefore some prejudice against synovectomy (figure 4.4).

Chemical agents

In Europe, and particularly in Scandinavia, osmic acid is extensively used, being sometimes com-

TABLE 4.1 SOME ISOTOPES USED FOR INTRA-ARTICULAR THERAPY

Isotope	Half-life (days)	Emission	Maximum energy of β (MeV)	Range in soft tissue (mm)		Range in cartilage (mm)	
				Mean	Maximum	Mean	Maximum
Erbium(^{169}Er)	9.5	β^-	0.34	0.3	1.0	0.2	0.7
Gold(^{198}Au)	2.7	β^-, γ	0.96	1.2	3.6	0.9	2.7
Rhenium(^{186}Re)	3.7	β^- (γ)	0.98	1.2	3.6	0.9	2.7
Yttrium(^{90}Y)	2.7	β^-	2.2	3.6	11.0	2.8	8.5

bined with steroid to minimise the inflammatory reaction (Martio *et al.*, 1972). Animal experiments have shown that osmic acid can produce damage to both articular and epiphyseal cartilage (Menkes *et al.*, 1972).

Physical agents: radiation and radiomimetic substances

Direct deep X-ray irradiation has been attempted and abandoned because it damages articular cartilage. Alkylating agents and radioactive colloids have also had extensive trials; their use in children is not advocated because of genetic risks, damage to articular and epiphyseal cartilage and the longterm risk of malignancy. Numerous trials have been carried out in adults using a great variety of materials. One of the earliest was thiotepa, an alkylating agent, and many papers have appeared on this substance and also on methotrexate and nitrogen mustard. The latter perhaps should be abandoned; the others, while less destructive, also produced an unacceptable degree of articular cartilage damage, and mutagenic and cellular toxic effects (Gristina *et al.*, 1970).

The radioactive colloids in common use were reviewed in a comprehensive symposium (Gumpel, 1973). These materials are β-ray emitters and their effect is essentially superficial. There is some γ-radiation from the gold colloid ^{198}Au which has led to its replacement by ^{186}Re(rhenium). Also in use are ^{169}Er(erbium) and ^{90}Y(yttrium). Lymphatic spread is dependent on colloidal size but to obtain an even irradiation of the tissues small particles are an advantage. Unfortunately, apart from ^{198}Au, with its disadvantages, no great

homogeneity of particle size is possible. Table 4.1 shows some of the characteristics (Ingrand, 1973). The colloid upon which the isotope is carried may influence its retention in the joint. Thus yttrium can be carried on ferric hydroxide, citrate or resin colloids. Although there has been much improvement in the safety of the materials used, the longterm effects on articular cartilage and the organism as a whole are unknown, as even with the 'safest' substance, radioactivity can be detected in lymph nodes and liver. Pre-medication with intra-articular steroid to reduce inflammation, combined with post-injection immobilisation, will reduce the risk of isotope spread. Chromosomal damage with mutagenic and neoplastic consequences, particularly leukaemia, are real hazards, particularly to the young. Hence, a whole-body dose of 10 rad increases the chance of cancer in a child but not in adults of 50 years.

Cryo-irrigation synovectomy

The known anti-inflammatory effect of cooling and the known differential tissue resistance to very low temperatures (Immamaliev, 1969) have led Chen and Helal (1977) to a trial of very low temperature irrigation of joints, firstly in normal rabbits and secondly in a rabbit model of rheumatoid synovitis. The results have encouraged a clinical trial of cryo-irrigation synovectomy.

Double osteotomy

Osteotomy above and below the knee joint results in reduction of synovial swelling considerably greater than that achieved by rest and immobilisation alone and probably occurs as the outcome

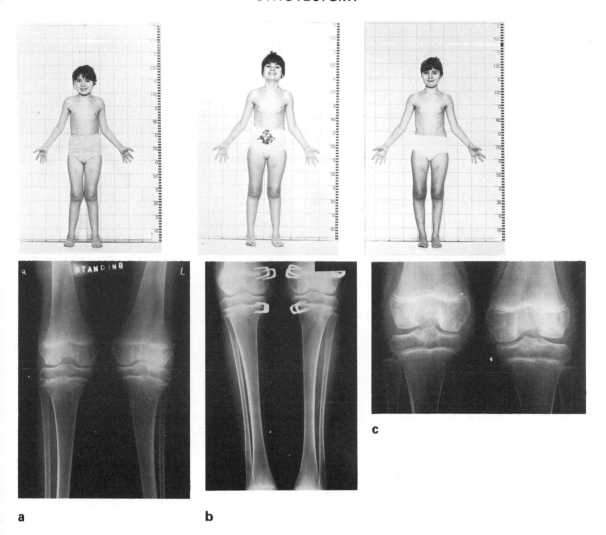

Figure 4.5 (a) Valgus knees; (b) treated by stapling; (c) slightly overcorrected staples removed (B. Ansell)

of an alteration in the synovial blood supply (Benjamin, 1969).

Surgical synovectomy

The knee joint

In children, particularly in synovectomy of the knee joint, it may be necessary to combine the operation with epiphyseal stapling to slow down overgrowth or to correct accompanying valgus deformity (figure 4.5). Reports suggest that anterior synovectomy suffices but Pahle (1975) recommends both anterior, and through a separate incision, posterior synovectomy. Brattström and Brattström (1972) combine osmic acid with surgical synovectomy, averaging a 70 per cent good result at 4 years. The osmic acid is injected intra-articularly some 2 weeks before operation.

Popliteal and calf cysts, as previously noted, will only resolve after anterior synovectomy; isolated excision of these cysts invariably leads to recurrence (Jayson *et al.*, 1972). Elbow synovectomy as noted by Wilson, Arden and Ansell (1973) and other studies, confirm the clinical impression that this is a satisfactory procedure, especially when combined with radial head excision.

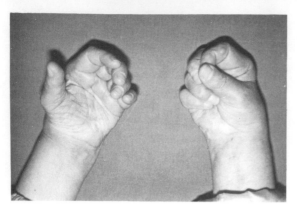

Figure 4.6 Synovitis within digital flexor sheaths grossly embarrasses flexing of left hand. Right hand has had synovial clearance with benefit

The wrist

Wrist joint synovectomy after excision of head of ulna is rewarding when the wrist joint is stable (Helal and Mikic, 1974).

Metacarpophalangeal and proximal interphalangeal joints

The metacarpophalangeal joints respond best if there are few erosions and the joints are stable. The interphalangeal joints do well provided they are free of fixed deformity.

Metatarso-phalangeal joints

Metatarsophalangeal synovectomy has been carried out on 18 feet in 11 patients. Pre-operatively all patients had pain and difficulty with walking unrelieved by insoles. All achieved complete pain relief. Post-operative follow-up is now from 8 months to 6 years. Four patients required further surgery within 3 years.

The ankle

Ankle synovectomies in two patients have not given satisfactory results.

The shoulder

Pahle (1973) reports eight patients, with a satisfactory outcome in the majority.

The hip

Of four patients, in whom anterior and posterior synovial clearance was carried out through separate approaches two remain well at 6 and 7½ years, respectively, and two have had replacement arthroplasties at 6 and 5½ years.

Tendon clearance

Wrist extensor synovectomy is rewarding both in terms of improved function and in prophylaxis against rupture. The carpal tunnel flexor synovectomy produces consistently good results in terms of function and relief of nerve compression symptoms. Decompression of the flexor apparatus over the metacarpal heads and within the digital flexor sheath (Helal, 1970, 1974) has realised excellent return of power and mobility in quite severely handicapped patients (figure 4.6). Decompression of tendons within the tarsal and peroneal tunnels has similarly resulted in a good clinical response.

CONCLUSION

Synovectomy is worthwhile and can provide long-term relief. The synovectomised joint may escape in generalised flares of the disease often for many years. Many Scandinavian surgeons perform synovectomy on quite badly damaged joints and will repeatedly synovectomise joints when the disease recurs. Much of so-called radiological deterioration may be based on a false premise, for if an immediate post-operative X-ray is taken, erosions not visible pre-operatively may be revealed and this X-ray state may remain stable for years. In practice, only a limited amount of synovium can be excised, yet this seems to provide a worthwhile response.

REFERENCES

Arthritis and Rheumatism Council & British Orthopaedic Association Report (1976). Controlled trials of synovectomy of the knee and metacarpo-phalangeal joints in rheumatoid arthritis. *Ann. Rheum. Dis.*, **35**, 437–442

Benjamin, A. (1969). Double osteotomy for the painful knee in rheumatoid arthritis and osteoarthritis, *J. Bone Jt Surg.*, **51B**, 694–699

Brattström, H. and Brattström M. (1972). Combined chemical and surgical synovectomy of the knee in rheumatoid arthritis, *Scand. J. Rheum.*, **4**, 101–102

Cassidy, J. T. and Boyle, G. G. (1966). Cutaneous atrophy secondary to intra-articular corticosteroid administration. *Ann. Intern. Med.*, **65**, No. 5, 1008–1018

Chen, S. C. and Helal, B. (1977). Personal communication

Gristina, A., Pace, N. A., Kantor, T. G. and Thompson, W. A. L. (1970). Intra-articular thio-tepa compared with depomedrol and procaine in the treatment of arthritis. *J. Bone Jt Surg.*, **52A**, No. 8, 1603–1610

Gumpel, J. M. (1973). Symposium on radioactive colloids in the treatment of arthritis. *Ann. Rheum. Dis.*, **32**, No. 6

Helal, B. (1970). Distal profundus entrapment in rheumatoid disease. *Hand*, **2**(1), 48–51

Helal, B. (1974). The reconstruction of rheumatoid deformities of the hand. *Br. J. Hosp. Med.*, 617–626

Helal, B. and Mikic, Z (1974). Ulnar head excision in the rheumatoid wrist, Paper read to *Rheumatoid Arthritis Surgical Society*

Immamaliev, A. S. (1969). The preparation, preservation and transplantation of articular bone ends. *Recent Advances in Orthopaedics*, Churchill, London, pp. 209–263

Ingrand, J. (1973). Characteristics of radioisotopes for intra-articular therapy. *Ann. Rheum. Dis.*, **32**, Suppl., 3–10

Jayson, M. I. V., St. J. Dixon, A., Kates, A., Pinder, I. and Coomes, E. N. (1972). Popliteal and calf cysts in rheumatoid arthritis. *Ann. Rheum. Dis.*, **31**, No. 1, 9–15

Martio J., Isomaki, H., Heikkola, T. and Laine, V. (1972). The effect of intra-articular osmic acid in juvenile rheumatoid arthritis. *Scand. J. Rheum.*, **1**, 5–8

Menkes, C. J., Piatier-Piketty, D., Zuchman, J., *et al.* (1972). Effets des injections articulaires d'acide osmique chez le lapin. Repercussion sur la croissance osseuse. *Rev. Rhum. Mal. Osteoartic*, **39**, 513–521

Pahle, J. (1973). Die synovektomie der proximalen interphalangeal gelenke. *Orthopäde*, **2**, 13–17

Pahle, J. (1975). Personal communication

Salter, R. B. and Murray, D. (1969). Effects of hydrocortisone on musculoskeletal tissues, *J. Bone Jt Surg.*, **51B**, 195

Wilson, D. W., Arden, G. P. and Ansell, B. M. (1973). Synovectomy of the elbow in rheumatoid arthritis. *J. Bone Jt Surg.*, **55B**, 106–111

5

OSTEOTOMY

Pain, deformity, synovial swelling and loss of function arising from joint damage due to rheumatoid disease may be relieved by osteotomy. Whereas correction of deformity was the original reason for osteotomy, the relief of pain and the dramatic reduction of swollen synovium at the knee, shoulder and metacarpophalangeal joints suggest that the mere division of bone, with its vessels and nerves, has a therapeutic effect. The sites where osteotomy may be indicated in rheumatoid disease include the spine, the lower jaw and the limbs (table 5.1).

THE EFFECTS OF OSTEOTOMY

(1) Pain relief.

(2) Correction of deformity.

(3) Regression of rheumatoid synovial swelling.

(4) Relative lengthening of contracted soft tissue.

(5) Improvement in X-ray appearance.

Pain relief

On awakening from anaesthesia, after osteotomy, patients frequently say that the arthritis pain has been replaced by discomfort associated with the wound. This observation, and the fact that pain is relieved in the non-weight-bearing joints of the upper limb, indicates a biological rather than a purely mechanical effect of osteotomy. Following successful osteotomy both clinical and radiological improvement may continue for 18 months.

Correction of deformity

Deformity may occur at joint level or in bone adjacent to the joint. Corrective osteotomy need not be exactly at the site of the deformity and it is well to consider the implications of this before operation. A compensatory correction is usually symptomatically satisfactory but may give rise to an unpleasant appearance such as the 'crank' deformity after correction of knee flexion contracture (figure 5.1). Full correction of valgus or varus deformity at the knee is desirable but residual deformity is consistent with many years of freedom from pain. Nevertheless persistent deformity

TABLE 5.1 OSTEOTOMY IN RHEUMATOID DISEASE

SITE	OSTEOTOMY	INDICATIONS
Spine	Cervical Lumbar	Deformity in ankylosing spondylitis
Jaw	Mandible, neck	To mobilise the temporomandibular joint in ankylosis and for pain in this joint in rheumatoid disease
	Mandible, body	To correct jaw deformity
Shoulder	Glenoid (Stamm) Double osteotomy	Acromial impingement Pain due to glenohumeral arthritis
Wrist	Lower end radius	Z and flexion deformity
Metacarpophalangeal	Double Oblique metacarpal	Painful synovitis Ulnar deviation and mobile swan-neck deformity
Hip	Intertrochanteric	Hip pain when rheumatoid process burned out.
Knee	Double	Painful synovitis with cartilage and bone damage accompanied by either valgus, varus, flexion or no deformity
	Supracondylar	Deformity, particularly valgus

	Upper tibial
	  high
	  low
	  Bracket
	  Gariepy
		Varus deformity

Metatarsal	Oblique 1st Oblique 5th Oblique 2nd–4th	Bunion Bunionette Claw toes and metatarsal head pressure

may contribute towards recurrence of symptoms due to unequal compartmental stress. Osteotomy at the knee should be planned in an effort to achieve a horizontal joint surface, for a more durable result can be expected from the even spread of load on the joint surfaces. Our results, surprisingly, do not always support this contention (figure 5.2). Whereas there is minimal latitude in the correction of valgus and varus deformity, there is none for knee flexion deformity, which should always be fully corrected.

Regression of rheumatoid synovial swelling

A hot, swollen, rheumatoid metacarpophalangeal joint rapidly subsides to normal size following osteotomies proximally and distally to the joint (figure 5.3). The reduction in joint swelling is dramatic and patients notice, within 10 days, that skin wrinkles, not seen for years, reappear and the shiny skin over their swollen joints resumes its normal appearance. A similar regression of synovium follows double osteotomy at the knee.

Relative lengthening of contracted soft tissue structures

The importance of relaxing soft tissues is not always fully appreciated. Thus varus intertrochanteric osteotomy produces a relative lengthening of muscles acting on the hip joint. In the hand, double osteotomy at the metacarpophalangeal joints shortens the bones and this can be increased by cutting of the metacarpals obliquely. If the obliquity is made such that the metacarpal head moves proximally and towards the ulnar side, those tight soft tissues causing ulnar deviation will be relaxed (figures 5.4 and 5.5). This operation

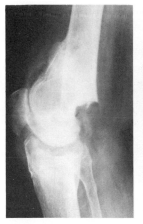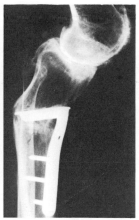

a   b

Figure 5.1 'Crank' deformity at the knee: (a) due to correction at the femoral osteotomy of knee flexion deformity; (b) a more severe 'crank' due to correction at a low tibial osteotomy far from the knee

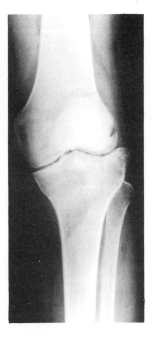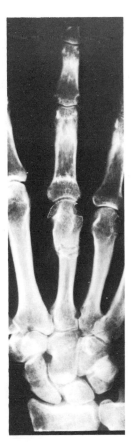

also corrects mobile swan-neck deformity due to intrinsic muscle contracture.

In the foot, oblique osteotomy of the first metatarsal (Wilson, 1963; Helal, Gupta and Gojaseni, 1974; Benjamin, 1975) slackens the taut, soft tissues which otherwise cause progression of hallux valgus deformity. In the presence of hallux rigidus, a wedge osteotomy at the base of the proximal phalanx, even in older patients, is preferable to arthrodesis, which, we feel, should be avoided in the first metatarsophalangeal joint. Oblique osteotomy of the 2nd–5th metatarsals not only relieves metatarsal head pressure in the sole, but also relaxes the long tendons which are causing progressive clawing (Helal, 1975); this operation has made excision of the metatarsal heads unnecessary in the majority of cases.

Left *Figure 5.2 X-ray taken in 1975 to show sloping joint surface in a knee which has remained entirely free from symptoms for 15 years after a double osteotomy in 1961 for burned-out rheumatoid disease*

Right *Figure 5.3 Double osteotomy of metacarpophalangeal joint. Note that the osteotomies are extraarticular*

Improvement in X-ray appearance

After successful osteotomy resulting in relief of pain there is often improvement in the X-ray appearance. The trabecular structure improves, bone density increases and, with the exception of the knee, the joint space widens and subchondral bone cysts resolve. These changes may result from increased joint activity consequent upon relief of pain and reversal of disuse atrophy.

SPINE

Spinal deformity is generally associated with ankylosing spondylitis. It is a good theoretical principle to correct at the site of the deformity (Simmons and Brown, 1972) but doubtful whether the risks of cervical and thoracic osteotomy, in the hands of most surgeons, are justifiable. The indication for surgery is limitation of forward vision, and if this can be corrected by lumbar osteotomy, then osteotomies in the dangerous cervical and

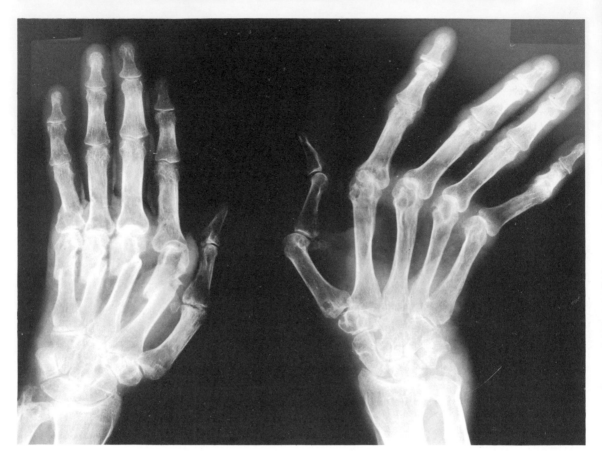

Figure 5.4 Double osteotomies of metacarpopha-langeal joints with oblique cuts of the metacarpals to correct ulnar drift. The most severely deformed of the two hands was operated on first

thoracic regions should be avoided. When the hips also are ankylosed in the flexed position, joint replacement of them generally removes the need for spinal osteotomy. Fracture of an ankylosed spine offers an opportunity to reduce the deformity; in the absence of neurological complications, bed rest, with appropriately placed pillows during union, permits a worthwhile degree of correction. It was in such circumstances that Smith-Petersen conceived the idea of spinal osteotomy (Smith-Petersen, Larson and Aufranc, 1945; Smith-Petersen, 1947).

union is prevented and the formation of a pseudarthrosis assured by the interposition of a silicone rubber block (Miller, Page and Griffiths, 1975; Ogus, 1977).

Osteotomy of the body of the mandible will correct dental malocclusion arising from disorders of mandibular growth in Still's disease.

JAW

Osteotomy of the neck of the mandible may relieve pain in adult rheumatoid disease, and in Still's disease and ankylosing spondylitis re-establishes lower jaw mobility. Following osteotomy, bone

SHOULDER

Osteotomy for rheumatoid disease in the upper limb relieves pain in a higher percentage of patients than osteotomy for pain in the lower limb. A double osteotomy of the glenoid neck and the

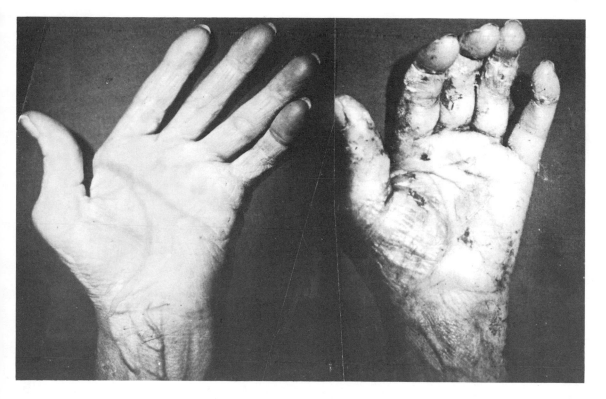

Figure 5.5 Before and after double osteotomy with oblique metacarpal cuts

surgical neck of the humerus without displacement dramatically relieves pain in rheumatoid disease of the shoulder (Benjamin, 1974; chapter 9). This relief is associated with considerable increase in total shoulder mobility. Sixteen patients subjected to double osteotomy were reviewed 1–7 years after operation (Benjamin, Arden and Hirschowitz 1977); 15 were improved, 12 of which had either slight pain or no pain. An early review of 13 subsequent operations reveals a similar result (chapter 9).

Displacement glenoid osteotomy (Stamm, 1963) may relieve acromial impingement. Its beneficial effect may be due to the osteotomy rather than the displacement.

WRIST

A wedge osteotomy of the radius, just proximal to the wrist, with its base situated dorsomedially has been described for flexion deformity of the wrist and Z deformity of the wrist and fingers. It is claimed that progression of ulnar deviation of the fingers is halted (Davison and Caird, 1976).

METACARPOPHALANGEAL JOINTS

Double osteotomy of the metacarpophalangeal joints relieves pain, reduces synovial swelling and improves grip strength. The indications are pain and swelling with consequent weakness of grip. The base of the proximal phalanx and the neck of the metacarpal are divided without opening the joint (figure 5.7). Fifty-five patients under our care have experienced this operation; of 37 reviewed 8–10 years later, 35 have remained free from pain, while 2 have recurrence of their synovitis. This operation is simple to perform (figure 5.8) and the post-operative regime merely consists of 10 days' immobilisation of the fingers by wool and bandage. The benefit is generally considerable; for example, most patients are able to lift a cup of tea or a teapot with one hand where

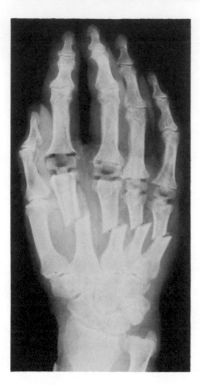

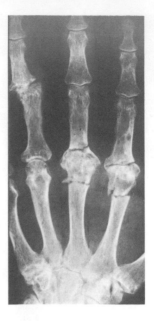

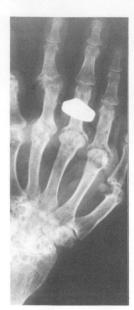

Figure 5.7 Double osteotomy of two metacarpopha-langeal joints immediately after operation (left) *and 3 years later* (right)

Figure 5.6 Swanson interposition arthroplasties with oblique metacarpal osteotomies to correct ulnar deviation

previously they required two. For ulnar deviation of the fingers we cut the metacarpal obliquely (figures 5.4 and 5.5) to relax the tight soft tissues. This may be combined with metacarpophalangeal joint arthroplasty (figure 5.6).

HIP

Although at present out of favour, intertrochanteric osteotomy has a place where the rheumatoid process is burned out and total replacement is contra-indicated (chapter 13).

KNEE

At the knee there is the choice either of a single tibial, a single femoral or a double osteotomy (Jackson and Waugh, 1961; Huskisson and Phillips, 1973; Coventry, 1965; Benjamin, 1969; Helal, 1962, 1965; Angel, Liyanage and Griffiths,

1974). However, the appropriate application of each type of osteotomy has not yet been ascertained. In degenerative arthritis with varus deformity, tibial osteotomy offers a high success rate, whereas with valgus deformity it does not (Harding, 1976; Coventry, 1975). Double osteotomy is equally rewarding in the presence of either varus, valgus or no deformity (Benjamin, 1976). Seventy-five per cent of our patients have their pain reduced by double osteotomy. Analysis of the 25 per cent of cases in which pain is not relieved does not reveal a constant factor but indicates which patients are most likely to benefit from the operation.

Favourable indications (Benjamin and Crabtree, 1977)

(1) Age below 70 years.
(2) Sero-negative.
(3) ESR less than 40 mm.
(4) No deformity.
(5) Absence of condylar collapse.
(6) Equal compartment disease.
(7) Not on long-term steroid therapy.

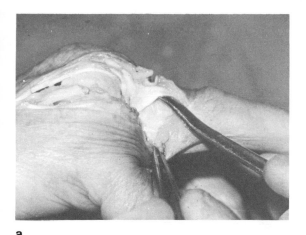

a

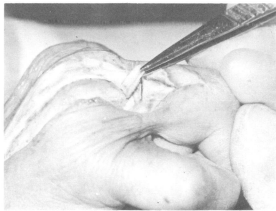

b

c

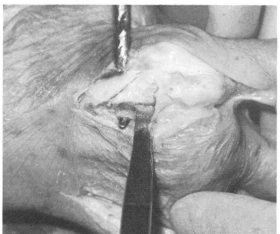

d

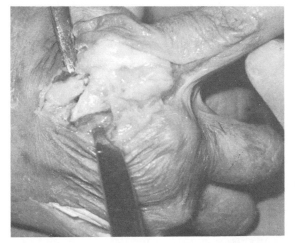

*Figure 5.8 Metacarpophalangeal double osteotomy:
(a) raising of the extensor hood to reveal the base of
the proximal phalanx; (b) the osteotomy of the
phalanx; (c) an oblique metacarpal cut; (d) telescoping in a proximal and ulnar direction of the
distal fragment*

After successful osteotomy, pain sometimes
recurs; this may be due to progression of the
rheumatoid process or to inadequate correction of
deformity. In a series of 74 double osteotomies for
knee pain, 60 were relieved of pain when assessed
2½–7 years after operation. When assessed at 10–
15 years post-operatively, 38 had remained free
from pain and in 22 the pain had recurred. Thus
half of the original series were still pain-free, and.

the 22 with recurrence of pain considered that 5–
15 years' freedom from symptoms had made the
operation well worth while. During those years
improved total knee prostheses were developed,
and as the patients were by then much older, they
entered a more suitable age group for replacement.

METATARSALS

Telescoping osteotomy of the metatarsals is
dramatically successful in relieving the painful
rheumatoid foot (chapter 15). Elevation of the
metatarsal heads following osteotomy relieves
localised pressure points in the sole, and the bone
shortening, with consequent relaxation of soft

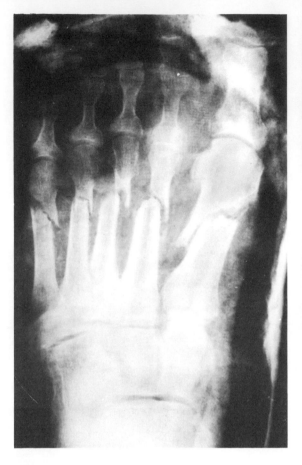

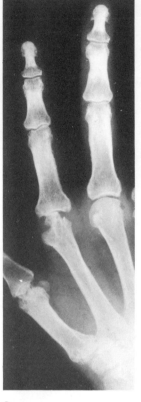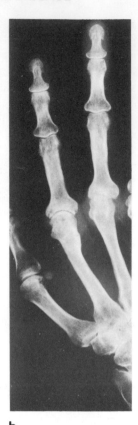

a   b

Figure 5.10 Metacarpophalangeal double osteotomy, index finger only: (a) immediately before operation in 1968; (b) 7 years later

Figure 5.9 Osteotomy of all five metatarsals, showing metatarsal head realignment

tissues, reduces mobile toe deformities and prevents the recurrence of fixed toe deformities previously corrected surgically. Osteotomy of all five metatarsals allows accurate realignment of the metatarsal heads (figure 5.9).

ACTION OF OSTEOTOMY

After the correction of deformity by osteotomy there is a change of weight-bearing stresses and strains, particularly with respect to articular cartilage. This alone may give pain relief but other mechanisms to account for the beneficial effects of osteotomy are likely. This is indicated by the following observations:

(1) Relief of pain may occur immediately post-operatively before the patient starts to weight-bear.

(2) Relief of pain in upper limb non-weight-bearing joints.

(3) Regression of rheumatoid hypertrophic synovium.

(4) Relief of symptoms in many patients in whom deformity at the knee is not corrected by operation.

Evidence suggests that venous tension is raised in the long bones adjacent to arthritic joints and that osteotomy reduces this intra-osseous pressure (Brookes and Helal, 1968; Arnoldi, Lemperg and Linderholm, 1971; figure 14.18, p. 187). These observations have inspired surgeons to devise operations to reduce intra-osseous pressure without osteotomy. The forage operation for the hip (Nissen, 1956), and drilling with the insertion of tubes as described by Arden and Hirschowitz (1976) are but two such procedures. Reduction in tibial intra-osseous pressure has been recorded following femoral osteotomy alone (Hirschowitz *et al.*, 1978).

During the months following osteotomy, X-ray changes are seen in the joints and the adjacent bone. These changes are not consistent but vary with the clinical result of the operation and with the joint involved. Following a clinically satisfactory osteotomy, there is an improvement in appearance of the X-ray with increased bone density (figure 5.10). X-ray translucency in rheumatoid disease is due not only to the inflammatory process, but also to disuse atrophy; the latter is reversed if pain is relieved and normal joint use regained. The stresses on weight-bearing joints are altered after displacement osteotomy and, as expected, there is rearrangement of the trabeculae. Regeneration of cartilage is known to occur following the Priddie (Priddie, 1959) procedure which consists of trephining degenerate articular cartilage and bone. Regeneration of articular cartilage may occur following osteotomy, thus accounting for the increase in joint space observed on X-ray. Joint movement is necessary for cartilage nutrition, and relief of pain leading to improved mobility encourages regeneration of cartilage.

GENERAL OPERATIVE TECHNIQUE

An oscillating saw or a pair of bone-cutting forceps is used for dividing the 2nd, 3rd and 4th metatarsal bones whereas an osteotome is preferable for the larger long bones. Heat necrosis and the precise cut which result from the use of the oscillating saw, predispose to non-union.

To osteotomise the shaft of a larger bone such as the femur, a series of 3-mm ($\frac{1}{8}$ inch) drill-holes is made along the desired cut (figure 5.11). A narrow osteotome is driven into the far cortex (figure 5.11b) and a broad osteotome is driven across the bone along the line of the drill-holes to meet the narrow osteotome already in place (figure 5.11c; cf. figure 13.4, p. 151). If osteotomy is attempted

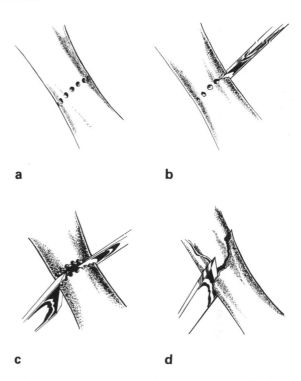

a   b

c   d

Figure 5.11 Osteotomy technique for the shaft of a long bone: (a) a series of 3 mm (⅛ inch) drill-holes in the line of the proposed osteotomy; (b) a narrow osteotome cuts the far cortex; (c) a broad osteotome is driven from the near cortex to meet the narrow osteotome; (d) splintering due to incorrect use of a single osteotome

using one osteotome alone, there is a danger of the bone splintering and of a spike from the distal cortex (figure 5.11d) preventing easy displacement of the osteotomy should it be desired.

Internal fixation

At the knee, internal fixation is seldom needed but when required a staple is generally adequate.

The Wainwright (1970) spline offers sufficient fixation for intertrochanteric osteotomy and allows the bone surfaces to settle together in the post operative days (figure 13.5, p. 152). We believe compression apparatus increases the danger of bone necrosis and also the compression plate may hold the bone surface apart, encouraging non-union. A previous displacement intertrochanteric osteotomy does not significantly add to the

64064

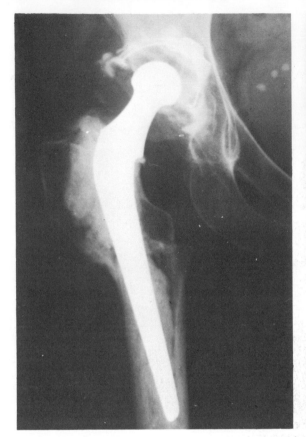

Figure 5.12 *Reformation of the medullary cavity by bone remodelling after a displacement osteotomy has made possible a subsequent total hip replacement*

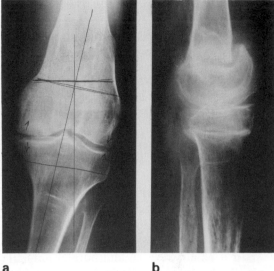

a   b

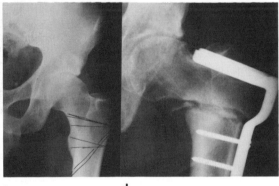

c   d

Figure 5.13 *Incorrect osteotomy: (a) a deformity-correcting wedge has been drawn on the X-ray. A wedge is unnecessary and the osteotomy although in the joint is not sufficiently distal; (b) the consequent non-union; (c) another wedge; (d) the consequent non-union*

technical difficulties of a total hip replacement or increase the morbidity provided the spline has previously been removed. After displacement, bone remodelling ensures a patent medullary cavity enabling the stem of a femoral prosthesis to be passed down the femur without undue difficulty (figures 5.12 and 13.26).

Wedges

It is a common practice to correct angulation by the removal of bone wedges. This is generally unnecessary. It increases the technical difficulty of the operation and predisposes to non-union (figure 5.13). In the rheumatoid patient deformity is corrected without difficulty by manipulation which compresses the bones on one side of the osteotomy and separates them on the other (figures 14.7 and 14.11, pp. 175 and 180).

TOTAL REPLACEMENT OR OSTEOTOMY

A careful appraisal of the patient is necessary (table 5.2). The risk of mechanical prosthetic

TABLE 5.2 TOTAL REPLACEMENT OR OSTEOTOMY AT THE KNEE

Age	Total prosthesis is undesirable under 60 years of age if osteotomy is a reasonable alternative.
Life expectancy	Osteotomy is contra-indicated unless more than 5 years.
Physical activity of patient	An active patient is liable to overstrain the prosthesis or its interface with bone.
Obesity	Obesity prejudices the results of all procedures especially knee replacement.
Condition of bone adjacent to joint	Good weight-bearing condylar bone is needed for osteotomy.
Corticosteroids	These prejudice the results of both procedures and, in particular, may increase the likelihood of loosening and infection of a prosthesis.
Activity of rheumatoid process	Local activity of the rheumatoid process is an indication for osteotomy at the knee, whereas it is a contra-indication at the hip.
Instability	Combined varus and valgus instability of the knee is a contra-indication for osteotomy and for those prostheses without intrinsic stability.
Severe fixed deformity	Valgus deformity may be an insuperable difficulty to prosthetic replacement, whereas double osteotomy corrects it with pain relief. Flexion deformity of over 35° is a contra-indication to osteotomy but is correctable by total replacement.
Loss of movement	Following osteotomy a few degrees of movement are always lost; consequently a useful range of movement is desirable if osteotomy is contemplated.
Skin condition	Varicose ulceration, psoriasis and other chronic skin conditions increase the probability of infection of a prosthesis.
Operating technique and theatre facilities	These must be of a high standard for total replacement surgery and a laminar flow ventilation system is desirable (chapter 6).

failure in a young active person is naturally higher than in an inactive elderly patient with a short life expectancy. The long post-operative recovery period required after osteotomy at a weight-bearing joint generally contra-indicates this operation in the elderly. The catastrophic complications of total replacement and the lesser complications of osteotomy must be discussed with the patient and his family before surgery. Prosthetic replacement is undesirable in the presence of chronic varicose ulceration; and osteotomy might be indicated in such circumstances where it would not otherwise be considered. Obesity increases complications following joint replacement, especially at the knee, whereas the results of osteotomy in the obese are satisfactory. In our experience previous osteotomy does not prejudice subsequent prosthetic replacement either at the hip or knee. Indeed, at the knee, correction of deformity by osteotomy and increased bone density following osteotomy leaves more satisfactory bone stock for subsequent prosthetic replacement.

REFERENCES

Angel, J. C., Liyanage, S. P. and Griffiths, W. E. G. (1974). Double osteotomy for the relief of pain in arthritis of the knee. *Rheumatology and Rehabilitation*, **xiii**, No. 3, 109–111

Arnoldi, C. C., Lemperg, R. K. and Linderholm, H. (1971). Immediate effect of osteotomy on the intramedullary pressure of the femoral head and neck in patients with degenerative arthritis. *Acta Orth. Scand.*, 42, 454–455

Benjamin, A. (1969). Double osteotomy for the painful knee in rheumatoid arthritis and osteoarthritis. *J. Bone Jt Surg.*, **51B**, 694

Benjamin, A. (1974). Double osteotomy of the shoulder. *Scand. J. Rheum.*, **3,** 65

Benjamin, A. (1975). Review of 160 first metatarsal osteotomies. *The British Foot Soc. Meeting.* November

Benjamin, A. (1976). Double osteotomy for arthritis of the knee, shoulder and finger joints. Clinical Demonstration. *6th Combined Meeting Orth. Ass. Eng. Speaking World,* London

Benjamin, A., Arden, G. P. and Hirschowitz, D. (1977). The treatment of arthritis of the shoulder joint by double osteotomy. *Int. Rheum. Meeting,* San Francisco

Benjamin, A. and Crabtree, S. (1977). In preparation.

Brookes, M. and Helal, B. (1968). Primary osteoarthritis, venous engorgement and osteogenesis. *J. Bone Jt Surg.,* **50B,** 493–504

Coventry, M. B. (1965). Osteotomy of the upper portion of the tibia for degenerative arthritis of the knee. *J. Bone Jt Surg.,* **47A,** 984

Coventry, M. B. (1975). Tibial osteotomy for arthritis of the knee. *J. Bone Jt Surg.,* **57B,** 110

Davison, E. P. and Caird, D. M. (1976). Osteotomy of the radius in rheumatoid disease. *Br. Orth. Ass.,* Spring Meeting

Harding, M. L. (1976). A fresh appraisal of tibial osteotomy for osteoarthritis of the knee. *Clinical Orthopaedics and Related Research,* No. 114 223–234

Helal, B. (1962). Osteoarthritis of the knee. *M. Ch. Orth. Thesis,* Liverpool

Helal, B. (1965). The pain in osteoarthritis of the knee, its causes and treatment by osteotomy. *Post-Grad. Med. J.,* **41** (474), 172–181

Helal, B. (1975). Metatarsal osteotomy for metatarsalgia. *J. Bone Jt Surg.,* **57B,** 187–192

Helal, B., Gupta S. K. and Gojaseni, P. (1974). Surgery for adolescent hallux valgus. *Acta Orth. Scand.,* **45,** 271–295

Hirschowitz, D., Edwards, J., Arden, G. P., Hart, G. and Shea, J. (1978). The treatment of the painful knee by reduction of intraosseous hypertension. Paper read at combined meeting of Heberden and British Orthopaedic Research Societies, March

Huskisson, B. C. and Phillips, H. (1973). A controlled trial of double osteotomies for rheumatoid arthritis. *Rheumatology and Rehabilitation,* **xii,** 214

Jackson, J. P. and Waugh, W. (1961). Tibial osteotomy for osteoarthritis of the knee. *J. Bone Jt Surg.,* **43B,** 746

Miller, A. M., Page, L. Jr and Griffiths, C. R. (1975). Temporo-mandibular joint ankylosis. *J. Oral Surg.,* **33,** 792–803.

Nissen, K. I. (1956). Personal communication

Ogus, H. D. (1977). Personal communication

Priddie, K. H. (1959). A method of resurfacing osteoarthritic knee joints. *J. Bone Jt Surg.,* **41B,** 618

Simmons, E. H. and Brown, M. E. (1972). Surgery for kyphosis in ankylosing spondylitis. *Can. Nurse.,* **68,** May, 24–29

Smith-Petersen, M. N. (1947). Personal communication

Smith-Petersen, M. N., Larson, C. B. and Aufranc, O. E. (1945). Osteotomy of the spine for correction of flexion deformity in rheumatoid arthritis. *J. Bone Jt Surg.,* **27,** 1

Stamm T. T. (1963). A new operation for chronic subacromial bursitis. *J. Bone Jt Surg.,* **45B,** 207

Wainwright, D. (1970). Upper femoral osteotomy. Robert Jones lecture. *Br. Orth. Ass.,* Autumn Meeting

Wilson, J. N. (1963). Oblique displacement osteotomy for hallux valgus *J. Bone Jt Surg.,* **45B,** 552–556

6

ARTHROPLASTY

Reconstruction by arthroplasty restores function and mobility to joints incapacitated by pain, deformity and limitation of movement. Arthroplasty may be achieved by the excision of bone-ends with or without the interposition of flexible material, by the grafting of articular cartilage and by total or partial prosthetic replacement.

Excision arthroplasty
Total
Elbow
Metatarsophalangeal joint (Fowler, 1959)
Interphalangeal joint (toes)
Partial
Lateral end of clavicle
Medial end of clavicle
Glenoid
Head of humerus
Head of radius
Distal end of ulna
Base of thumb metacarpal
Trapezium
Proximal row of carpal bones
Heads of metacarpals
Head and neck of femur
Patella

Heads of metatarsals (Kates, Kessel and Kay, 1967)
Bases of proximal phalanges of toes

Interposition arthroplasty
Autogenous
Prosthetic

Replacement by autogenous cartilage graft
Perichondrial graft for interphalangeal joint

Replacement by homologous cadaveric allograft
Partial
Total

Replacement by prosthesis
Partial
Total

EXCISION ARTHROPLASTY

Total

Elbow

Complete excision may be indicated for a severely damaged rheumatoid elbow or for retrieving the situation should a total prosthesis fail. Bone excision must be generous to enable the resulting space to fill with fibrous tissue giving some stability as well as movement. However, the stability achieved is often insufficient for good function, and this procedure is only contemplated as a last resort.

Metatarsophalangeal joint

Fowler's operation, consisting of the excision of both metatarsal heads and the bases of the proximal phalanges, has been superseded in our practice by metatarsal osteotomy, except in cases of severe foot deformity associated with considerable skin ulceration, when bone excision allows skin healing by relief of tension.

Interphalangeal joint

In the feet, simple excision of the proximal or distal interphalangeal joints is generally sufficient to correct deformity. After excision, the distal joints are held in position by skin sutures and recurrence of flexion is prevented by tenotomy of the long flexor tendon; the proximal interphalangeal joints may be held straight for 3 weeks by a Kirschner wire to enable fibrous union to develop. A spike arthrodesis is more appropriate than excision in the case of the proximal interphalangeal joint of the second toe.

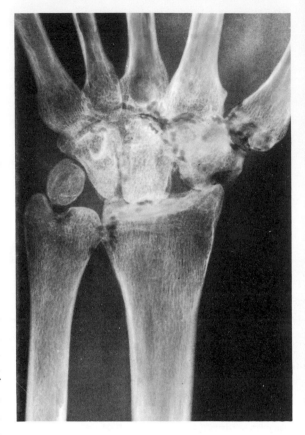

Figure 6.1 Excision of the proximal row of carpal bones

Partial

The lateral and medial ends of the clavicle

Painful disease of the acromioclavicular and the sternoclavicular joints is generally relieved by an injection of hydrocortisone and local anaesthetic; if this fails, then either end of the clavicle may be excised.

Glenoid

Glenoidectomy is recommended by Wainwright (1974) and Gariepy (1976).

Head of humerus

Excision of the head of the humerus is only mentioned to be condemned, for more effective

and less mutilating procedures are available (chapter 9).

Head of radius

Excision of the head of the radius, often combined with synovectomy, gives lasting relief for the painful elbow (Wilson, Arden and Ansell, 1973; chapter 10).

Distal end of ulna

Excision of the distal 15 mm ($\frac{5}{8}$ inch) of ulna relieves wrist pain due to disease or subluxation of the lower radioulnar joint. For extensive wrist disease distal ulna excision is combined with either fibrous stabilisation of the wrist or arthrodesis.

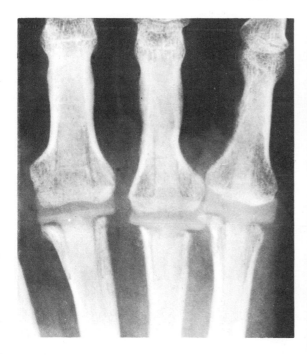

Figure 6.2 Swanson metacarpophalangeal spacer prostheses

Base of thumb metacarpal

We prefer to excise the trapezium for arthritis at the base of the thumb.

Trapezium

Excision of the trapezium, for painful arthritis at the base of the thumb, results in surprisingly little disability, even in patients who require a firm hand grip for work or sport.

Proximal row of carpal bones

Excision of the trapezium, lunate and scaphoid bones through a transverse dorsal incision is a technique which is cosmetically acceptable and results in excellent function. The appearance of a wrist so treated is such that even on careful observation and palpation it is difficult to credit the removal of these three bones (figure 6.1).

Heads of metacarpals

The excision of one or more metacarpal heads, in metacarpophalangeal disease, relieves pain and

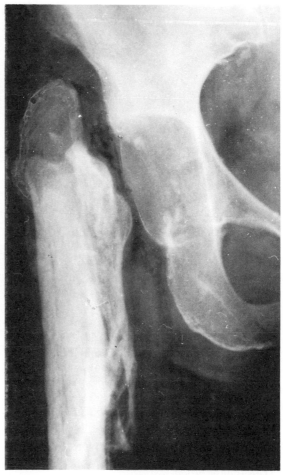

Figure 6.3 Girdlestone excision anthroplasty

corrects deformity; it is now common practice to add a silicone rubber prosthesis between the metacarpal and the proximal phalanx to act as a spacer (Swanson, 1973; Nicolle and Calnan, 1972; figure 6.2). Neither excision of the metacarpal heads nor insertion of metacarpophalangeal silicone rubber prostheses will prevent recurrence of deformity, for it is necessary to realign tendons and release contracted soft tissue.

Head and neck of femur

Girdlestone (1943) excision arthroplasty (figure 6.3) of the hip is a remarkable operation for considerable stability as well as mobility follows removal of the head and neck of the femur

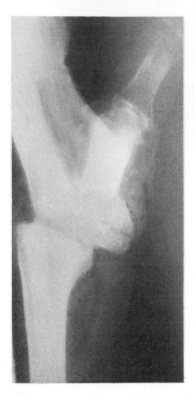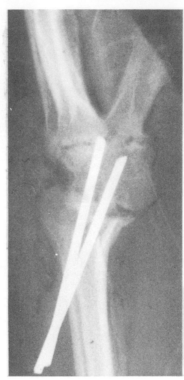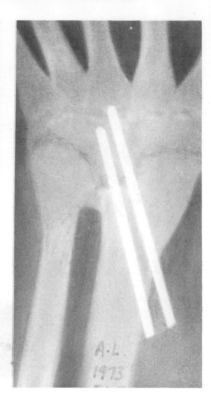

Figure 6.4 Fibrous stabilisation of the wrist with correction of palmar subluxation (E. Lance)

too, has been largely replaced by metatarsal osteotomy.

provided meticulous post-operative care is undertaken (chapter 13).

Patella

It is tempting in severe patellofemoral disease to remove the patella; unfortunately the pain relief seldom lasts and this, added to other disadvantages of patellectomy, far outweigh any benefit.

Heads of metatarsals

Prominent metatarsal heads causing pain in the sole of the foot can be excised but, in our practice, osteotomy of the metatarsal necks has largely replaced this procedure.

Bases of proximal phalanges of toes

Excision of the bases of the proximal phalanges of the toes, including Keller's procedure for the hallux, is no longer part of our usual practice; it

INTERPOSITION ARTHROPLASTY

Autogenous

After surgical mobilisation of a joint, by a more or less extensive excision of diseased tissue, bony ankylosis may be prevented by the interposition of autogenous fascia. For example, the dorsal capsule may be interposed between the lower end of the radius and the proximal row of carpal bones (Colwell, 1976; Stellbrink and Tillman, 1976) and stabilisation achieved by temporary internal fixation with crossed Steinman pins after removal of diseased tissue and correction of displacement (Lance, 1976; figure 6.4). This produces an acceptable firm, fibrous ankylosis at the wrist where movement is not vital. Good results of autogenous interposition arthroplasty are claimed by Campbell, Kimura and Vainio, both at the elbow and at the knee (Campbell, 1921, 1922; Kimura and

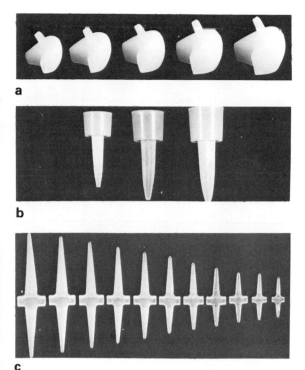

Figure 6.5 Silicone rubber spacers (A. Swanson): (a) lunates; (b) heads of radius; (c) metacarpophalangeal joints

Vainio, 1976). We prefer to interpose a silicone membrane at the elbow in the rare cases where this is indicated; we have had no personal experience of its insertion at the knee joint.

Prosthetic

Sheets of plastic material interposed between the bone-ends are generally no more satisfactory than sheets of fascia, whereas various designs of silicone rubber prosthesis do prevent ankylosis and maintain joint mobility. Silicone rubber spacers have been designed for the wrist and elbow joints and silicone rubber prostheses for replacing small bones and the ends of long bones (Swanson, 1973; figures 6.5 a and b). Silicone rubber metacarpophalangeal joint prostheses act not only as spacers, but also as flexible hinges and internal moulds around which a new joint capsule forms

(Swanson, 1973; figure 6.5c). At the hip joint the interposition of a cup (Smith-Petersen, 1939; Adams, 1953) to prevent bony union between the femur and acetabulum has been superseded by various designs of total joint replacement.

REPLACEMENT BY AUTOGENOUS CARTILAGE GRAFT

Autogenous perichondrium from a costochondral junction is grafted to the bone-ends of damaged small joints in the hand; it is claimed that new cartilage is formed by the grafted perichondrium (Enqvist, 1976).

REPLACEMENT BY HOMOLOGOUS CADAVERIC ALLOGRAFT

Partial

Osteochondral allografts are incorporated by the host without immunosuppression; these allografts have been used to replace bone and cartilage in unicompartmental degenerative disease in the knee as well as in spontaneous osteonecrosis. The early results are encouraging and the technique may in time prove of value in rheumatoid disease (Gross *et al.*, 1976; chapter 14; figure 14.20).

Total

The massive replacement with cadaveric knee joints is generally followed by tissue rejection; despite isolated successes, this technique at present has no practical application (Imamaliev, 1969; Laurence, 1976).

REPLACEMENT BY PROSTHESIS

A prosthesis not only provides one or more articulating surfaces, but also acts as a spacer preventing apposition of the bone-ends and consequent fibrous or bony union.

Partial

The articulating surface of a partial prosthesis articulates with the undisturbed cartilage of the opposing joint surface. In rheumatoid disease, as both joint surfaces are generally damaged, the partial prosthesis has only a limited place in treatment. At the hip, replacement of the femoral head alone is unsatisfactory, as the acetabulum, damaged by disease, is inadequate as a bearing surface and central dislocation of the prosthesis follows.

At the shoulder, replacement of the head of the humerus (Neer, 1958) is not associated with undue wear of the glenoid cavity, as the shoulder is not a weight-bearing joint. Nevertheless replacement of the humeral head is not part of our practice, as the shoulder is relieved by less mutilating procedures (chapter 9).

The Platt prosthesis (figure 14.21, p. 188), a metal covering for the femoral surface of the knee joint, has been superseded by the more versatile MacIntosh tibial plateau prosthesis (MacIntosh, 1967), which can replace both tibial articular surfaces independently. By selecting the prosthesis of appropriate thickness, valgus, varus and flexion deformity may be corrected (see figure 14.22, p. 189); Kates has modified the prosthesis and cements it into the tibia.

Many partial excision arthroplasty techniques as described above may be completed by inserting a silicone rubber prosthesis. However, removal of the trapezium, excision of the head of the radius and excision of the lower end of the ulna are so successful on their own that generally these implants are unnecessary. Keller's procedure may be enhanced by a silicone rubber replacement for the base of the proximal phalanx. As an alternative a silicone rubber spacer, similar to that used in metacarpophalangeal joint replacement, may be inserted between the first metatarsal and the proximal phalanx (Whalley and Wenger, 1975; chapter 15).

Total

Total joint prostheses have been developed for all of the major and several of the minor synovial

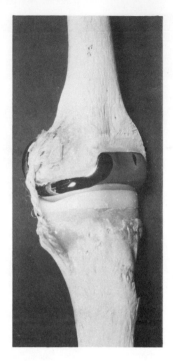

Figure 6.6 Freeman–Swanson knee (M. Freeman)

joints of the skeleton. Their success is often due to the co-operation between surgeon and biomechanical engineer. Despite this success, research into rheumatoid aetiology and possible prevention of joint destruction must not be diverted by the discovery of a solution of the end phase, namely the replacement of joints. Biomechanical enthusiasm has to be tempered by a predominantly clinical approach which gives priority to the patient's needs.

Upper limb

Total prosthetic replacement of the larger joints of the upper limb is at present unrewarding. Several shoulder prostheses have been designed but the problem of reproducing rotator cuff function remains, for total abduction of the shoulder of over 90° is seldom achieved.

The humerus and ulna do not provide adequate anchorage for the fixation of an elbow prosthesis and consequently hinged joints loosen. This problem may be overcome by the development of unconstrained prostheses (Institute of Mechanical Engineers, 1977; chapter 10).

Lower limb

Hip

The history of prosthetic replacement of the hip joint, dating back to 1885, was reviewed by Scales in 1967. The success of prosthetic hip joints is due to their ball-and-socket design and to the low frictional qualities of the materials used in manufacture. Movement can take place in every plane with consequently comparatively little torsional force on the bone—cement interface, which would otherwise fail more frequently with consequent loosening of the prosthesis.

Knee

Many designs of total knee prosthesis have, and are being, developed (Institute of Mechanical Engineers, 1977) but the problem of prosthetic simulation of human knee function is considerable. In order to provide stability, some constraint is necessary between the femoral and tibial surfaces; however, such constraint between these articular surfaces leads to the transmission of forces, particularly torque to the bone—cement junction, predisposing to loosening. The early knee prostheses were hinged, totally constrained with excellent stability but a high rate of loosening; their place in the treatment of rheumatoid disease is considerably limited.

The second generation of total knee prostheses are unconstrained (Freeman and Swanson, 1972; figure 6.6). The femoral component rests on the tibial-bearing, and as long as the ligaments are not destroyed by disease or damaged by the surgeon, and provided the plane of the joint is horizontal, these unconstrained prostheses can be satisfactory.

The third generation of prostheses are partially constrained; these have cemented intramedullary stems and allow some rotation, consequently reducing the likelihood of loosening (Attenborough, 1974; Sheehan, 1974).

Whereas a good prosthetic hip will allow strenuous activity, there is no prosthetic knee which should be put to similar stress. A good prosthetic knee is suitable for negotiating stairs, sitting, standing and walking, but that is all. The post-

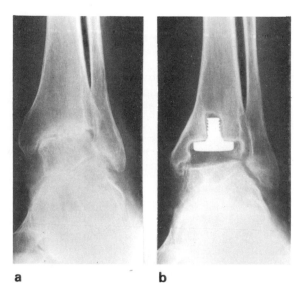

a   b

Figure 6.7 (a) Rheumatoid disease in the ankle (J. Kirkup); (b) Smith ankle replacement (J. Kirkup)

operative recovery period following total knee replacement is short, and there is consequently pressure upon the surgeon to insert such prostheses too early when a stable knee would benefit perhaps from an osteotomy, a procedure liable to fewer and less serious complications.

Ankle

An efficient ankle prosthesis will prove of great value as the forces thrown upon the foot joints after ankle arthrodesis are excessive. Ankle prostheses are at present too early in their development for general use but they show promise (Smith, 1977; Kirkup, 1977; figure 6.7).

Foot

Peritalar joint dysfunction may be remedied by a variety of prostheses now under development. The lateral stop and talonavicular prosthesis are two of these (chapter 15; figure 6.8). These prostheses are experimental and none has yet replaced triple arthrodesis.

TOTAL PROSTHETIC JOINT REPLACEMENT AFTER OSTEOTOMY

In our experience, osteotomy at either the hip or the knee does not prejudice subsequent total prosthetic replacement provided there is sound bony union. At the knee, correction of deformity by osteotomy facilitates subsequent total knee replacement, as varus or valgus deformity would add to the technical problems encountered. At the hip, bone plates, splines and screws from the internal fixation of a previous osteotomy should be removed at least 3 months before total replacement. When such apparatus is removed at the time of total replacement, post-operative complications increase. Following an intertrochanteric osteotomy, even when considerably displaced, the process of bone modelling reforms a continuous medullary cavity (see figure 13.26), so permitting reaming and placement of the femoral component. In the rare event of difficulty due to central callus, reaming is facilitated by first drilling the medulla with the guidance of a Read jig (Read, 1969; figure 13.27, p. 164).

POST-OPERATIVE COMPLICATIONS OF PROSTHETIC JOINT REPLACEMENT

These can be summarised as follows:
Infection
  Early
  Late
Skin flap necrosis
Metal sensitivity and toxicity
Cement toxicity
Loosening
  Failure of technique
  Steroids
  Undue physical activity
  Infection
Fat embolus
Dislocation
Mechanical failure
  Cement
  Metal
  Plastics
  Bone

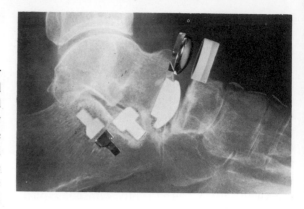

Figure 6.8 Talonavicular and lateral stop prostheses

Ectopic calcification
Thrombophlebitis
Later complications
Surgery after failure
  Removal of prosthesis and cement
  Revision
  Excision arthroplasty
  Arthrodesis

Infection

Deep infection is catastrophic for the patient and extremely worrying for the surgeon. In the hip and knee the prostheses generally have to be abandoned, and even after their removal with the cement, infection may be difficult to eradicate. Some patients still have discharging sinuses at their death, which has been hastened by the infection (Hunter and Dandy, 1977; Poss *et al.*, 1976).

Early infection, within 1 month of surgery, is likely to be due to wound contamination in the operating theatre. However, infection may be introduced into the depths of the wound by retrograde spread along suction drainage tubes. There is some doubt as to the value of these tubes and they should be removed within 24 hours of operation. Desquamating psoriasis and chronic varicose ulceration increase the probability of infection. Urinary tract infection and blood-borne infection of the hip or knee may follow urethral catheterisation (Donovan, Gordon and Nagel, 1976; Barrington and Wright, 1930). In recent years there has been an alteration in hospital bacterial flora, and penicillin-resistant organisms such as *Pseudomonas* and *Enterobacter* are occasionally found to be the pathogens in deep hip infection. Infection by these organisms will diminish if anti-staphylococcal antibiotics are given for no longer than 3 days and if catheterisation is avoided during the early post-operative period.

Late blood-borne infections may occur many years after operation, the organism often being identified with those of a concurrent infection such as a sore throat, a skin infection or a dental abscess (Downes, 1977). When dental surgery is undertaken in a patient with a prosthesis, antibiotic cover is given, and root fillings are best avoided in rheumatoid disease (chapter 1). Antibiotic cover is advisable not only in the presence of dental sepsis, but also whenever there is a clinical infection with a possibility of bacteraemia.

Prevention of infection

A meticulous regimen is necessary. In the wards, patients for total prosthetic replacement should be isolated from others with known infection and preferably admitted not more than one or two days before operation, to reduce the probability of contamination by resistant hospital organisms. Operation is only undertaken if there is no focus of infection, including even the smallest skin pustule. Perineal, finger and nasal swabs are incubated and the growth of a pathogenic organism is an indication to delay surgery and start antiseptic bathing. Preferably the operating theatre is reserved solely for orthopaedic patients and it should lie fallow for at least a day on two occasions in the week. This has the dual purpose of allowing pathogenic organisms to die and of giving the staff adequate theatre cleaning time. Laminar flow ventilation and a body-exhaust system are recommended but the Charnley–Howarth tent is probably unnecessary. There should be minimal movement or talking in the theatre and no unnecessary persons present. Perhaps the most important single item is that the surgeon and his assistants wear two pairs of operating gloves, the outer pair being changed during surgery—for example, on each occasion before handling cement. Operating gowns and drapes for the patient should be impermeable. Trousers should be worn by both male and female members of the staff and should be close-fitting or tied at the ankles to reduce skin-shedding. We give 1 g of cephaloridine intravenously at the commencement of the anaesthetic; 1 g is given 6 hours post-operatively and 1 g 12 hours post-operatively; thereafter a cephalosporin is given by mouth for 3 days only. Either gentamycin, cephaloridine or Fucidin is mixed with the cement (Buchholz and Gartmann, 1972; Elson *et al.*, 1977; table 6.1) and the wound is irrigated during the operation with noxythiolin (Horsfield, 1967), an effective antibacterial agent against Gram-negative bacteria.

Skin flap necrosis

It is at the knee that skin flap necrosis must be avoided. Care is taken to protect the skin by reflecting with it as much deep tissue as possible to ensure its blood supply (Sheehan, personal communication). To prevent skin necrosis (figure 6.9) we now use a midline skin incision so long as there is no previous parapatellar scar. The capsule is incised medially. Allgover Basle or subcuticular sutures reduce strangulation of skin, which may occur with other sutures. Owing to poor blood supply of the wound margin, a small area of skin necrosis sometimes occurs at the level of tibial tuberosity (see figure 14.16, p. 186); this heals spontaneously if there is an underlying osteotomy but is a potential source of danger in the presence of a prosthesis. Where the viability of the skin edge is in doubt knee flexion is delayed until the skin is healed.

Metal sensitivity and toxicity

The significance of tissue sensitivity is ill-understood, for a patient whose skin reacts to a metal may have deep tissues which do not. Consequently skin sensitivity found during the investigation of a patient with a loose prosthesis may or may not be significant. Such sensitivity may have arisen after the insertion of the prosthesis, and the value of pre-operative skin sensitivity tests is uncertain.

Stainless steel and cobalt – chrome metal-on-metal prostheses release microparticles which can cause local fibrosis and in the knee may strangulate the overlying skin (figure 6.10). The metal can be found throughout the body and there is said to be a danger from the carcinogenic action of cobalt, although there seems to be little evidence to support this suggestion.

Cement toxicity

Monomer has toxic properties. The quantity of unfixed monomer reduces as mixed cement becomes firmer during setting; consequently the later it is inserted the less monomer is free and the less likely it is to cause toxicity. On removal of the tourniquet after the insertion of a total knee prosthesis free monomer may be rapidly distributed into the general circulation. Sheehan advises the operating table be tilted 30° head down before the tourniquet is released and a careful watch kept on the blood-pressure. The monomer is a vasodilator and adequate blood volume must be maintained. Monomer may be a hazard to theatre staff and unnecessary handling of setting cement with bare hands should perhaps be avoided. After setting, particles of cement can damage the plastic component of the prosthesis and care is taken to remove these by means of a curette, forceps or irrigation before the components are reduced.

Loosening

Diagnosis

The diagnosis of loosening of a prosthesis is not always easy; however, pain is generally the pre-

TABLE 6.1 SOME PRECAUTIONS TO PREVENT PROSTHETIC INFECTION

In the ward

Patients admitted within one or two days of operation to prevent contamination by hospital bacteria.
Some ward beds to lie fallow to allow opportunity for ward-cleaning.
Ward flower vases frequently changed and sterilised.
Ward curtains frequently changed and cleaned.
Antiseptic bath on day before and day of operation.
Iodine skin preparation if not sensitive.
The appointment of a control-of-infection sister with the support of a microbiologist in order to monitor infection, observe possible sources of infection and regularly swab staff for carriers of pathogenic organisms.
Full investigation of patient to find and eradicate foci of infection.
Prostatectomy if there is danger of urinary retention which might necessitate catheterisation.

In the theatre

Staff with infective foci excluded.
Education of theatre nursing and medical staff, including itinerant junior medical staff, in proper scrubbing-up and aseptic techniques.
Redline procedure at door of theatre.
Ward beds not allowed in theatre.
Redline around operating table within which no one but the surgeon and immediate assistants are allowed.
No unnecessary movement of personnel in theatre.
No unnecessary talking by personnel in theatre.

No unnecessary conversation between personnel within and outside theatre.
Operating theatre for clean orthopaedic patients only.
Overoperating avoided in theatre.
Fallow weekend and one day in the week.
Two masks.
Two pairs of gloves, second pair changed after draping and after each cement mix.
Care with cuffs where sweat from the surgeon's forearm may penetrate the gown (Charnley, 1976).
Non-permeable wrap-around disposable gowns.
Trousers worn by male and female theatre staff, tight-fitting at the ankle or tied there to prevent skin shedding.
Non-permeable disposable drapes.
Gentle handling of tissues (Laurence, 1977).
Dead space obliterated by vertical sutures to prevent haematoma.
Suction drainage trochar-spigot left attached to the tube until the moment it is ready for connection to the vacuum bottle.
Monofilament nylon or wire for skin suture, otherwise totally buried subcuticular suture.

Post-operation

No ward dressing.
If blood soaks through theatre dressing, a sterile pack immediately placed over the original dressing and strapped to the skin as organisms traverse wet dressings.
Suction drainage discontinued within 24 h of surgery.
Avoid catheterisation.

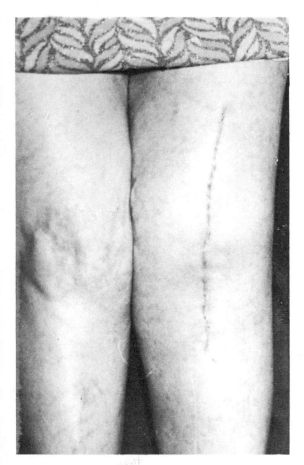

Figure 6.9 *Straight midline anterior incision for exposure of the knee joint*

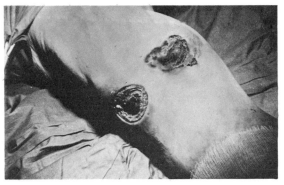

Figure 6.10 *Skin necrosis 1 year after an apparently successful total knee replacement. The subcutaneous tissues down to the prosthesis were impregnated with particles of metal surrounded by avascular fibrous tissue*

Failure of technique

Early loosening of the acetabular component of a total hip prosthesis can follow inadequate removal of soft tissue from the acetabulum and lack of keying due to a too smooth surface. Two or three keying-holes, approximately 12 mm ($\frac{1}{2}$ inch) across, drilled into, but not through, the pelvic bones, are advised and several 3-mm ($\frac{1}{8}$ inch) drill-holes made with a protected drill. The medullary cavity of the long bones should be reamed out thoroughly and care taken that cement extends beyond the tip of the prosthetic stem. At the upper end of the femur the cancellous tissue in the great trochanter is removed with a Volkmann's spoon so that cement extends to the cortex, which is better able to take load than cancellous bone. Inadequate bony covering of the acetabular component may also result in its loosening. McKee's method of building up a buttress of cement with two keying screws helps to deepen the bony socket, but such build-up either of the femoral or of the acetabular areas in order to seat the prosthetic components may be a prelude to future trouble. It is better to extend the roof of the acetabulum by taking a bone block from the femoral head and fixing it to the ilium (Harris *et al.*, 1977).

Steroids

The decalcification characteristic of rheumatoid disease is made worse by steroid therapy and

senting feature. Radiologically a narrow band of translucency may surround the cement, although this also occurs without symptoms and its significance is doubtful. Obvious movements of the prosthesis may take place and be seen on X-ray with or without screening. Arthrography with radio-opaque material is sometimes diagnostic and is conducted under the X-ray screen, preferably with the patient anaesthetised and relaxed. Distraction by an axial pull on the limb allows radio-opaque material to pass between the cement and bone, this space may otherwise be occluded by muscle tension. Nevertheless the radio-opaque fluid also enters this interval in some symptom-free patients.

increases the probability of loosening of all prosthetic components.

Undue physical activity

Loosening of a total prosthesis which had previously been satisfactory sometimes occurs following a single injury such as a fall downstairs, for the cohesion at the interface between cement and bone will fail if the stresses applied to it are too great. After a knee prosthesis the patient should be advised to limit his or her activity to gentle walking. The risk of a knee prosthesis loosening also increases with the added stresses consequent upon obesity. Hip prostheses are able to take greater stresses and strains, yet it is difficult to advise a patient to what extent he or she should curtail sporting activities. The majority of rheumatoid patients are restricted by multiple joint damage such that they cannot take part in violent sport. Running or jarring should be avoided and thus soccer is not advised for any patient after a total hip prosthesis, whereas gentle family badminton may do no harm. Non-competitive tennis on grass courts rather than hard may be harmless and a good skier who is unlikely to fall may ski provided he or she limits their activities to the easier runs and avoids soft snow. Most orthopaedic surgeons have patients with total prostheses taking part, without trouble, in strenuous sporting activities, but a few such examples do not justify indiscriminate activity, as any increase in stress will increase the probability of loosening and prosthetic failure.

Infection

Whenever loosening of a prosthesis is suspected, full investigation to exclude infection should be carried out. A technetium or gallium radioisotope scan is of value in making this diagnosis (chapter 3) but it is sometimes difficult to be certain whether infection is present or not, even after an exploratory operation.

Fat embolus

A narrow plastic tube should be placed in the medulla of long bones while the cement is inserted,

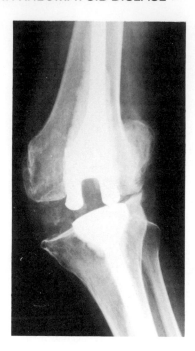

Figure 6.11 Subluxation of a Sheehan knee

to prevent the build-up of increased medullary pressure which may initiate fat embolus. The use of a cement syringe also prevents this increase in pressure.

Dislocation

Early dislocation following hip prosthesis occurs most commonly as the result of faulty technique. A frequent cause of dislocation is misalignment of the acetabular and femoral components. It is essential that with the leg lying at rest the femoral head points directly into the acetabulum and is neither significantly anti- nor retroverted. Attempts to correct external rotational deformity are frequently unsuccessful and predispose to dislocation. It is preferable to accept this deformity rather than prejudice stability.

It is inadvisable to replace a hip joint if there is fixed flexion deformity of more than 30° in the knee on the same side. Such deformity predisposes to dislocation of the hip and should be corrected before the hip operation.

The Howse snap-fit prosthesis (figure 13.14, p. 155) is intended to reduce the likelihood of dis-

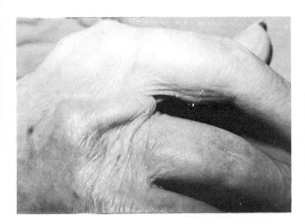

Figure 6.12 Dislocation of a Swanson metacarpo-phalangeal prosthesis from the phalanx. The patient was delighted with the result and did not wish further surgery

location, especially in the early post-operative period.

The prosthetic hip is in danger of dislocation during the move from the operating-table to the recovery area and from there to the ward. After a posterior approach an abduction wedge (see figure 13.29a, p. 164) is applied before the patient's transfer to the trolley and after an anterior approach the feet may be bandaged together to prevent external rotation (see figure 13.29b). This bandage is kept in place until the patient awakens fully. Dislocation probably occurs more readily after a posterior approach, following which, sitting should be avoided completely for 1 week and confined to a high chair for the following 3 weeks. During the first week the patient should be restricted to either lying flat or else standing in order to avoid hip flexion.

In the ward the bed table is placed so that any movement of the patient towards it will internally rotate the replaced hip if an anterior approach was used, and externally rotate the hip if a posterior approach was used (see figure 13.30, p. 165).

If the prosthesis is thought to be unstable at operation an abduction pillow is used with the patient remaining in bed for 3 weeks. In the event of early dislocation, closed reduction under anaesthesia is usually possible, and if the hip is held abducted for three weeks, it generally becomes stable. Cast bracing allows early mobilisation (see p. 165).

For stability, unconstrained knee prostheses require intact ligaments and a horizontal joint line. If the joint line is not horizontal, there is a tendency for the femur to slide off the tibia. This has been observed in an incorrectly inserted Freeman–Swanson knee (figure 14.25b, p. 190): it is sometimes difficult to ensure precise positioning of this prosthesis. Partially constrained knee prostheses are usually sufficiently stable to prevent dislocation although the Sheehan knee can sublux (figure 6.11) and dislocate.

Silicone rubber metacarpophalangeal joints may dislocate from the metacarpal or proximal phalanx (figure 6.12).

Mechanical failure

Cement

The temperature of storage, the temperature at the time of use and the efficiency of mixing are considered critical when acrylic cement is used in industry. In operating theatre technique there is no standardisation of storage temperature and no standardisation of temperature at time of use, and, compared with industrial methods, the mixing of powder and monomer is inefficient. The consistency of the cement when inserted into the bone varies from site to site, from summer to winter and from surgeon to surgeon. Barium and antibiotics may be added to the cement, and such additions vary the physical characteristics of the cement. If the modulus of elasticity is significantly different from that of bone, bending and torsion may break down the interface between cement and bone. Standardisation of these variables of temperature, mixing, additions and time of insertion may improve cement characteristics (Lee *et al.*, 1977).

Metal

After return to full activity, stems of the femoral prostheses sometimes fracture (see figure 13.37); thus strengthened prostheses have been designed for use in heavy patients. These fractures sometimes occur near the tip of the stem.

Plastics

Wear of the high-density polyethylene seldom causes prosthetic failure.

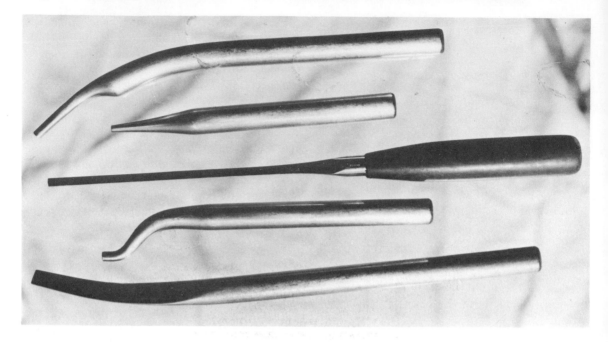

Figure 6.13 Instruments to remove cement from the shaft of the femur without de-roofing

Bone

The shaft of the femur sometimes fractures near the tip of the femoral prosthesis. Fortunately, it is usually unnecessary to revise the prosthesis, as the fracture often unites if immobilised. Any difficulty with this treatment demands the insertion of a long-stem femoral prosthesis; in the future the Chichester straps and plates (Partridge, 1977; see figure 13.32, p. 166), although not yet perfected, may become a satisfactory alternative.

Ectopic calcification

See chapter 13.

Thrombophlebitis

See chapter 13.

Later complications

In any series of total prostheses a number of cases of late loosening, fracture and infection occur each year. Careful follow-up of such series is necessary to assess the significance of these later complications. In the case of the hinged knee prostheses, the greater the body weight the sooner in the post-operative years does the prosthesis loosen.

Surgery after failure of prosthesis

Removal of prosthesis and cement

For failure of the arthroplasty it is usually desirable to remove the prosthesis and the cement. To remove cement from long bones is never easy and it may be necessary to de-roof the medullary cavity. When revision is contemplated, de-roofing is undesirable and can be avoided with specially designed instruments (figure 6.13) in the case of the femoral shaft, by cutting a small cortical window near the distal extremity of the cement and hammering the cement proximally, and alternating this with the use of the long narrow osteotome inserted into the medullary cavity from the neck of the femur. The Read jig (figure 13.27) enables the femur to be drilled correctly despite the cement. Even a small hole in the cortex weakens the femoral shaft, which may fracture; thus a long-stem femoral component is advisable for the

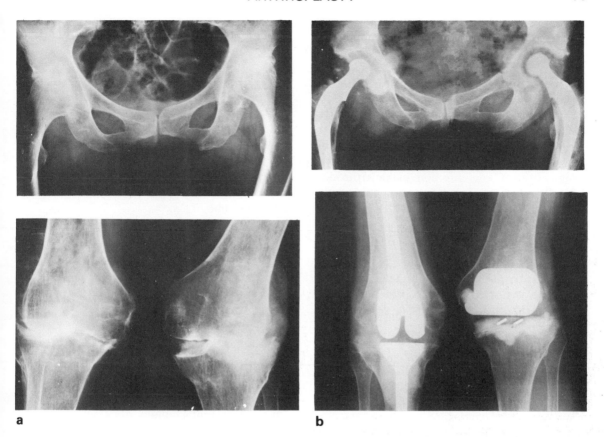

a   b

Figure 6.14 Total joint replacement of both hips and both knees: (a) before replacement—both hips severely damaged and extremely painful. Both knees also damaged and painful after 5 and 6 years' freedom from pain after double osteotomies; (b) total prosthetic replacement of the hips—Freeman–Swanson knee on the left and a Sheehan knee on the right. All are at present painless and mobile after 6, 4 and 2 years, respectively

revision. During the insertion of the acetabular component a plug of cement may penetrate the pelvis. The central drill-hole which allows this is generally not necessary in rheumatoid disease, where the thin floor of the acetabulum seldom has to be reamed. The Charnley expanding reamer, modified by the removal of the centring knob, is suitable for any reaming required. If the floor of the acetabulum is pierced, then the-hole should be occluded by a 'Mexican Hat' cement restricter and every effort made to prevent cement entering the pelvis, as its later removal may be difficult.

Revision

After loosening of a prosthesis without infection or after fracture of one of the components, revision may be undertaken. Revision is usually more difficult technically than the primary operation and is associated with a higher rate of complication. The early supposition that a worn prosthesis can easily be replaced must now be modified in the light of the complication rate of such procedures. Revision of a total prosthesis for infection requires courage. Buchholz uses a mixture of cement and gentamycin, and his results are encouraging (Buchholz and Gartmann, 1972).

Excision arthroplasty

This is a most successful line of retreat for the hip, as the fibrosis of previous surgery provides stability for the Girdlestone operation. The efficacy of excision arthroplasty is dependent upon meticulous post-operative care aimed at achieving abduction and neutral rotation (chapter 13). Excision arthroplasty is the only choice after removing an unsuccessful elbow prosthesis.

Arthrodesis

It is particularly important in the design of a total knee prosthesis that its removal should ensure that sufficient cancellous bone remains in both the femur and the tibia to permit arthrodesis without undue shortening of the lower limb. A poor design, cement and infection make arthrodesis difficult and fibrous ankylosis may be the best that can be achieved (see figure 14.31a, p. 196). The consequent disability can be considerable and permanent external splintage may have to be worn (figure 14.31b).

CONCLUSION

A rheumatoid patient confined to bed and racked with pain can be transformed by arthroplasty (figure 6.14). Careful selection to match the surgical technique with the patient and the disease is the keystone of success.

REFERENCES

Adams, J. C. (1953). A reconsideration of cup arthroplasty of the hip with a precise method of concentric arthroplasty. *J. Bone Jt Surg.*, **35B**, (2), 199

Attenborough, C. G. (1974). Total knee replacement using a stabilised gliding prosthesis. *Conference on Total Knee Replacement*, Inst. Mech. Eng.

Barrington, F. J. F. and Wright, H. D. (1930). Bacteraemia following operations on the urethra. *J. Path. Bact.*, **33**, 871–888

Buchholz, H. W. and Gartmann, H. D. (1972). Prevention of infection and operative management of insidious deep infection in total endoprosthesis. *Chirurg*, **43**, 446–453

Campbell, W. C. (1921). Arthroplasty of the knee. *J. Orth. Surg.*, **3**, 430

Campbell, W. C. (1922). Arthroplasty of the elbow. *Ann. Surg.*, **76**, 615

Charnley, J. (1976). *Br. Med. J.*, Dec. 25

Colwell, J. C. (1976). Arthroplasty of the wrist in rheumatoid arthritis. *Rheum. Arth. Surg. Soc. Meeting.*, Toronto

Donovan, T. L., Gordon, R. O. and Nagel, D. A. (1976). Urinary infections in total hip arthroplasty. *J. Bone Jt Surg.*, **58A** (8), 1134–1137

Downes, E. M. (1977). Late infection after total hip replacement. *J. Bone Jt Surg.*, **59B** (1), 42–44

Elson, R. A., Jephcott, A. E., MeGechie, D. B. and Veretas, D. (1977). Bacterial infection and acrylic cement in the rat. *J. Bone Jt Surg.*, **59B** (4), 452–457

Enqvist, O. (1976). Reconstruction of joint cartilage with free perichondrial graft. *Hand Society Meeting*

Fowler, A. W. (1959). Method of forefoot reconstruction. *J. Bone Jt Surg.*, **41B**, 507

Freeman, M. and Swanson, S. A. V. (1972). *J. Bone Jt Surg.*, **54B**, 170

Gariepy, R. (1976). Glenoidectomy in the repair of the rheumatoid shoulder. *6th Combined Meeting Orth. Ass. Eng. Speaking World*, London

Girdlestone, G. R. (1943). Acute pyogenic arthritis of the hip. Operation giving free access and effective drainage. *Lancet*, **i**, 419

Gross, A. E., Langer, F., Haupt, J., Pritzher, K. and Friedlander, G. (1976). Allotransplantation of partial joints in the treatment of osteoarthritis of the knee. *Clin. Orth.*, **108**, 7–14

Harris, W. H., Crothers, O. and Oh, I. (1977). Total hip replacement and femoral-head bone-grafting for severe acetabular deficiency in adults. *J. Bone Jt Surg.*, **59A** (6), 752–759

Horsfield, D. (1967). *In vitro* studies of the action of noxythiolin on antibiotic-resistant Gram-negative bacteria. *Clin. Trials J.*, **4** (1), 625–628

Hunter, G. and Dandy, D. (1977). The natural history of the patient with an infected total hip replacement. *J. Bone Jt Surg.*, **59B** (3), 293–297

Imamaliev, A. S. (1969). The preparation, preservation and transplantation of articular bone ends. *Recent Advances in Orthopaedics*, Churchill, London, pp. 209–263

Institute of Mechanical Engineers (1977). *Joint Replacement in the Upper Limb*, Mechanical Engineering Publications, London

Kates, A., Kessel, L. and Kay, A. (1967). Arthroplasty of the forefoot. *J. Bone Jt Surg.*, **49B,** 382

Kimura, Ch. and Vaino, K. (1976). Arthroplasty of the elbow in rheumatoid arthritis. *Arch. Orthop. Unfall-Chir.*, **84,** 339–348

Kirkup, J. (1977). Personal communication

Lance, E. (1976). Fibrous stabilisation of the wrist. *Rheum. Arth. Surg. Soc. Meeting.* Toronto

Laurence, M. (1976). Transplantation of articular cartilage. *Rheum. Arth. Surg. Soc. Meeting* Toronto

Laurence, M. (1977). A surgeon's respect for the skin. *Wld Med.* January

Lee, A. J. C., Ling, R. S. M., Vangala, S. S. and Buck, S. (1977). Some clinically relevant variables affecting the mechanical behaviour of bone cement. *Br. Orth. Ass.* Autumn Meeting

MacIntosh, D. L. (1964). Arthroplasty of the knee in rheumatoid arthritis using the hemiarthroplasty prosthesis. In: *Synovectomy and Arthroplasty in Rheumatoid Arthritis: Second Int. Symp.* (ed. G. Chapchal), Thieme, Stuttgart

Neer, C. S. (1958). Shoulder prosthesis. *J. Bone Jt Surg.*, **40A,** 960

Nicolle, F. V. and Calnan, J. S. (1972). New design of finger prosthesis for the rheumatoid hand. *Hand*, **4,** 135

Partridge, A. (1977). Nylon plates and straps for internal fixation of osteoporotic bone. *Lancet*, **ii,** April 9, 80

Report of the working party in acrylic cement in orthopaedic surgery. (1974). Submitted to the DHSS

Poss, R., Ewald, F. C., Thomas, W. H. and Sledge, C. B. (1976). Complications of total hip replacement arthroplasty in patients with rheumatoid arthritis. *J. Bone Jt Surg.*, **58A** (8), 1130–1133

Read, J. (1969). Hertford. Personal communication

Scales, J. T. (1967). Arthroplasty of the hip using foreign materials: a history. *Symposium on Lubrication and Wear in Living and Artificial Human Joints*, Institute of Mechanical Engineers

Sheehan, J. M. (1974). Arthroplasty of the knee. *Conference on Total Knee Replacement*, Institute of Mechanical Engineers

Sheehan, J. M. Typed instructions for insertion of prosthesis. Personal communication

Smith, R. C. (1977). Smith total ankle procedure. Issued by manufacturer (Wright and Co. Ltd). Reported at *Am Orth. Ass. Meeting*, Las Vegas

Smith-Petersen, M. N. (1939). Arthroplasty of the hip. A new method. *J. Bone Jt Surg.*, **21,** 269

Stellbrink, G. and Tillman, K. (1976). Resektion-interposition arthroplastik des Handgelenks bei der chronischen Polyarthritis. *Verh. Dtsch. Ges. Rheum.*, **4,** 530–534

Swanson, A. B. (1973). *Flexible Implant Resection Arthroplasty in the Hand and Extremities*, Mosby, St. Louis

Wainwright, D. (1974). Glenoidectomy. A method of treating the painful shoulder in severe rheumatoid arthritis. *Ann. Rheum. Dis.*, **33,** No. 1, 110

Whalley, R. C. and Wenger, R. (1975). Total replacement of the first metatarsophalangeal joint. *J. Bone Jt Surg.*, **57B**

Wilson, D. W., Arden, G. P. and Ansell, B. M. (1973). Synovectomy of the elbow in rheumatoid arthritis. *J. Bone Jt Surg.*, **55B,** 1

7
ARTHRODESIS

When adjacent joints remain painless and mobile, arthrodesis of a major joint may be compensated for satisfactorily, whereas it may cause severe disability in progressive rheumatoid disease. In the lower limb an arthrodesed joint may become an insuperable barrier to rising from a chair, and in the upper limb it may inactivate an otherwise useful hand.

Arthrodesis may be indicated in the spine, the ankle, the wrist, the tarsus and some of the smaller joints. It is the treatment of choice in disease of the distal interphalangeal joints and the metacarpophalangeal joint of the thumb, and is the best salvage procedure for an infected knee prosthesis.

A successful arthrodesis relieves pain, corrects deformity and gives stability. While this consequent functional improvement may allow the contralateral limb to be spared, the disadvantages of arthrodesis in rheumatoid disease far outweigh the advantages except in certain situations. In the years following an arthrodesis, compensatory movement in neighbouring joints aggravates the rheumatoid process, increasing joint destruction and instability. This is often seen in the foot following an ankle arthrodesis and in the neck at either end of an arthrodesed section (figure 7.1).

CERVICAL SPINE

Instability of the cervical spine associated with increasing neurological signs, unrelieved by traction or a plaster cast, is an indication for fusion of the unstable joints, and is best confined to as short a segment as possible. Instability may be in an anteroposterior direction, commonly a forward movement of the atlas on the axis, or a vertical subluxation of the odontoid process into the foramen magnum (chapter 8). In either case sudden death may supervene but in neither case is the radiological appearance alone an absolute indication for surgery. Neurological changes frequently improve or remain unaltered without treatment or with simple immobilisation. Even vertical odontoid subluxation is compatible with many years of freedom from symptoms (figure 7.2). The risks of surgery for cervical instability have to be weighed against the possible increase of neurological damage with non-operative measures.

SHOULDER

During the past 8 years only 12 patients were recommended for surgery for shoulder pain due to

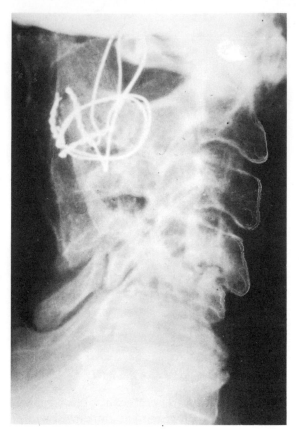

Figure 7.1 Aggravation of rheumatoid disease at the lower end of a fused section of cervical spine with consequent subluxation

removed many indications for arthrodesis (chapter 9).

ELBOW

Arthrodesis of the elbow is difficult to achieve and the resulting disability outweighs any advantages; consequently it is not recommended.

WRIST

Arthrodesis of the wrist by the insertion into the carpus of a wedge fashioned from the distal end of the radius after Brockman (Nissen, 1951; figure 7.3) or by the Mannerfelt method (chapter 11) is a simple and successful procedure. Although relieving pain and offering stability, wrist arthrodesis is seldom needed owing to the success of synovectomy combined with excision of the lower end of the ulna (Helal and Mikic, 1973). Even in the presence of palmar subluxation of the carpus, fibrous stabilisation (chapter 6) is often sufficient to give the patient a stable painless wrist with some mobility (chapter 11).

CARPOMETACARPAL JOINT OF THE THUMB

Simple excision of the trapezium relieves the pain of carpometacarpal rheumatoid disease without significant loss of function; consequently arthrodesis, which is quite difficult to achieve at this site, is rarely indicated. It has been claimed that arthrodesis offers more thumb stability and so may be advised in the heavy-manual worker. There is little evidence to support this claim, and generally patients with rheumatoid disease are not in heavy industry.

METACARPOPHALANGEAL JOINT OF THE THUMB

The normal range of movement of this joint varies from 5° to over 90° and its arthrodesis is not

glenohumeral rheumatoid disease, whereas in the same period 344 rheumatoid knees were subjected to surgery. Until recently the only operation available to relieve the severe pain of glenohumeral arthritis was arthrodesis, and in view of the magnitude of the operation, and its disabling effects, the rheumatologist hesitated to refer his patient to the surgeon. The operation is technically difficult, requires several months' immobilisation in a plaster of Paris spica cast, and is not always successful. The loss of all glenohumeral movement, particularly rotation, increases the difficulty of combing the hair and adjusting clothing at the back. If arthrodesis of the shoulder is advised, then a compression technique with a lag screw may be used. Fortunately the relief of pain following double osteotomy of the shoulder has

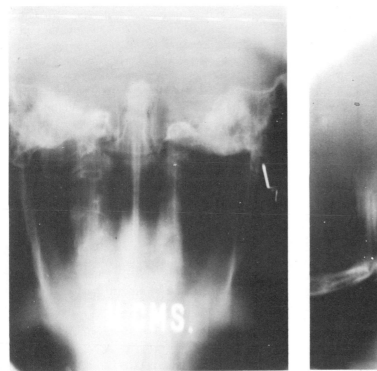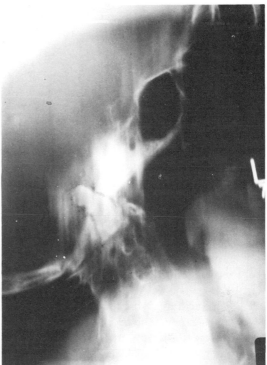

Figure 7.2 Tomograms to show the odontoid process which is often difficult to see on straight films. There is considerable upward displacement of the odontoid through the foramen magnum. There were no signs of neurological damage even though conservative treatment only was given. Operation was contra-indicated for other reasons

Figure 7.3 Wedge arthrodesis of the wrist

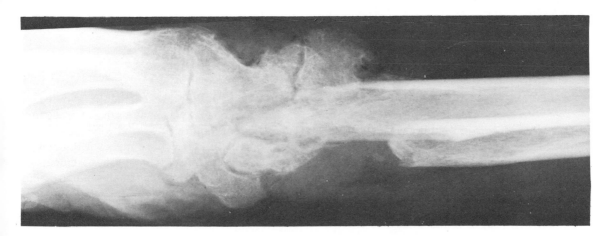

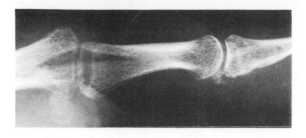

Figure 7.4 Harrison–Nicolle peg arthrodesis of the metacarpophalangeal joint of the thumb

associated with significant loss of function. In those cases of thumb deformity where secondary mobile flexion or extension of the interphalangeal joint exists, the functional benefit from fusion of the metacarpophalangeal joint alone is remarkable. Fusion of this joint as well as fusion of the interphalangeal joints of the thumb and fingers have been facilitated by the Harrison–Nicolle polypropylene peg (Harrison, 1977). The operation to insert it is simple and the painless fibrous union observed at 6 weeks generally converts to firm bony union in 12–18 months (figure 7.4).

INTERPHALANGEAL JOINT OF THE THUMB

An index thumb pinch-grip made ineffective by instability of the thumb interphalangeal joint is restored by arthrodesis. Fusion of both the interphalangeal and metacarpophalangeal thumb joints is indicated when both are severely diseased.

PROXIMAL INTERPHALANGEAL JOINTS OF THE FINGERS

Prostheses and silicone rubber spacers have a limited place in rheumatoid disease of these joints. The problems due to porotic bone and attenuated articular and extra-articular soft tissue combine to thwart a return of useful function. When bone destruction is advanced and synovectomy unlikely to benefit, arthrodesis is indicated. The introduc-

tion of the Harrison–Nicolle peg has transformed this operation from a difficult, sometimes unsuccessful, procedure to an easy and generally satisfactory operation. The combination of arthroplasty of the metacarpophalangeal joints of the fingers with arthrodesis of the proximal interphalangeal joints results in good hand function, combining a desirable degree of mobility with stability.

DISTAL INTERPHALANGEAL JOINTS OF THE FINGERS

Instability and pain in these joints in collagen disease seldom justify surgery, but when symptoms are severe, the joints are best treated by arthrodesis.

THE HIP

Arthrodesis of the hip is not recommended in rheumatoid arthritis. The disease is often bilateral, and in the unlikely event of both hips being unsuitable for some form of reconstruction, bilateral Girdlestone excision arthroplasty is preferable to arthrodesis. In the female, arthrodesis of this joint interferes with sexual intercourse (Greengross, 1972; Harris and Currey, 1971; Currey, 1970).

THE KNEE

Arthrodesis of the knee should be avoided in rheumatoid disease except as a salvage procedure following the failure of a total joint prosthesis. Even one arthrodesed knee makes it difficult to travel by public transport and to sit in a cinema or theatre. The disease seldom remains monarticular and bilateral fused knees are a calamity, for the upper limbs are usually not strong enough to enable the rheumatoid patient to rise from a chair.

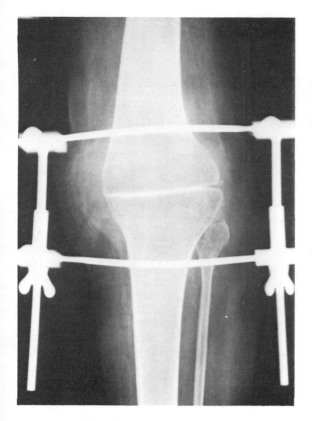

Figure 7.5 Charnley compression arthrodesis of the knee, not always advisable in rheumatoid disease because of the danger of bone collapse

Primary arthrodesis is technically easy in rheumatoid disease. Compression with clamps is inadvisable, as the skeletal pins may cut through the porotic bone and the soft subchondral bone may collapse under compression. Staples are simple to insert and offer a successful alternative (figure 7.5 and 7.6). Secondary arthrodesis after the removal of a failed prosthesis is difficult to achieve, even though the prosthesis may be specially designed to leave adequate cancellous bone for fusion (figure 14.31, p. 196).

THE ANKLE

Arthrodesis relieves pain and instability due to rheumatoid disease in the ankle but it throws undue stress on the subtaloid and midtarsal joints.

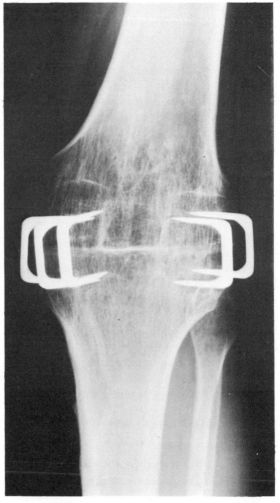

Figure 7.6 Arthrodesis of the knee using staples

As these joints are generally also diseased when the ankle is affected, they deteriorate more rapidly after ankle arthrodesis. It is hoped that a suitable ankle joint prosthesis will provide a satisfactory alternative.

SUBTALOID JOINT

A triple arthrodesis corrects deformity, stabilises the hind-foot and relieves pain in subtaloid and midtarsal rheumatoid disease. This arthrodesis does not generally aggravate disease in the ankle, because increased strain is thrown on the ankle joint only when walking on uneven ground, and subtaloid disease is often accompanied by a relatively normal ankle. When both the ankle and subtalar joints are diseased, a pantalar arthrodesis may be indicated. However, this can be a great handicap and one anticipates a successful ankle and subtalar prosthesis being developed for extensive hind-foot disease.

MIDTARSAL JOINTS

Isolated disease of the calcaneocuboid joint is uncommon, but if it occurs, it is simply treated by arthrodesis using staple fixation.

Disease of the talonavicular joint is generally an indication of strain on the joint and is frequently associated with subtalar disease; consequently the entire peritalar joint complex must be carefully examined. If the talonavicular joint alone is the seat of symptoms, it may be arthrodesed, but the implications must be carefully considered, as this fusion interferes with subtalar joint movements.

METATARSOPHALANGEAL JOINTS

This joint in the lateral four rays never requires arthrodesis and seldom needs it in the hallux.

PROXIMAL INTERPHALANGEAL JOINTS OF THE TOES

Spike arthrodesis is infrequently indicated in rheumatoid disease, since most patients present with metatarsalgia due to prominent metatarsal heads and the clawing is secondary. The introduction of oblique metatarsal osteotomies (chapter 15) combined with manipulative straightening of the toes by rupturing the plantar plate produces a satisfactory result. Following this procedure, the toe is splinted straight for 3 weeks with a Kirschner wire.

DISTAL INTERPHALANGEAL JOINTS OF THE TOES

The interphalangeal joint of the hallux may be arthrodesed using a Harrison–Nicolle peg, whereas the distal joints of the lateral four toes need only be excised and held extended by deeply placed skin sutures. If the distal joint is flexed, excision of the joint should be combined with tenotomy of the long flexor tendon to prevent recurrence.

REFERENCES

Currey, H. L. F. (1970). Osteoarthrosis of the hip joint and sexual activity. *Ann. Rheum. Dis.*, **29** (5), 488–493

Greengross, W. (1972). *Marriage, Sex and Arthritis*, Arthritis and Rheumatism Council

Harris, J. and Currey, H. L. F. (1977). Sexual problems due to disease of the hip joint.

Harrison, S. H. (1977). Stabilisation of the first metacarpophalangeal joint with straight Harrison–Nicolle pegs. A review of 100 cases. *Combined Meeting American and British Hand Societies*, Edinburgh

Helal, B. and Mikic, Z. (1973). Survey of ulnar head excision and synovectomy. *Mtg. Rheum. Arth. Surg. Soc.*

Nissen, K. I. (1951). Orthopaedic surgery in congenital spastic paralysis. *Proc. R. Soc. Med.*, **44**, 87

8

THE SPINE

In rheumatoid disease the spine is affected in three ways: by synovitis of the joints, by ligamentous damage and by bony destruction and collapse.

CERVICAL SPINE

The neck gives rise to most of the serious disability and surgical problems posed by rheumatoid involvement of the spine. Synovitis of the facetal joints gives rise to pain; this usually settles with general treatment of the disease and the provision of a collar. Intervertebral instability as a result of ligamentous damage is most commonly seen at atlanto-axial level (figure 8.1) and it is not uncommon to find evidence of instability on X-ray without symptoms. Movements of the odontoid process of the axis produce posterior impingement of the cord, and both mechanical and vascular elements contribute to cord damage. The first complaint is of suboccipital neck pain which radiates to the back of the head, while clinically, limitation of movement and diminution in the range of rotation occur early. Neurological involvement can range widely in severity between mild paraesthesiae in upper or lower limbs or both, and tetraplegia. In atlanto-axial displacements, neurological involvement may occur by direct compression or oedema, or by vascular spasm or occlusion of spinal cord vessels. Direct occlusion of the vertebral vessels may also take place. Rana *et al.* (1973) have analysed the important neurological findings and shown that the ophthalmic and maxillary divisions of the trigeminal nerve are often involved, as are the pyramidal tracts and the sensory pathways. Fasciculation is an early sign.

Whenever general anaesthesia is contemplated for the rheumatoid patient, the possibility of cervical spine damage must be borne in mind, for in the presence of subluxation, careless handling may produce severe spinal cord damage.

Signs of cervical spine instability

(1) Clunking: on flexion/extension a jerk is seen or felt.

(2) Palate sign: the index finger feeling the posterior pharyngeal wall can detect abnormal flexion/extension (Matthews, 1969; figure 8.2).

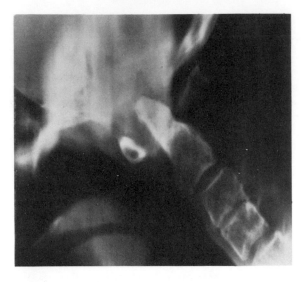

Figure 8.1 Subluxation at atlanto-axial level (note separation of odontoid process from arch of the atlas)

Figure 8.2 Through the open mouth the index finger is placed on the posterior pharyngeal wall. This demonstrates the possibility of palpating the gap between the arch of the atlas and odontoid process with the patient's head in flexion/extension

(3) With the patient lying supine, occiput on the thenar eminence of the examining left hand with the ring and little fingers on the spine of the axis and atlas, it is possible to detect relative movement between the atlas and axis on flexion/extension of the neck. We are against the use of this manoeuvre in the hands of the inexperienced as it may result in neurological damage.

(4) Cerebrospinal fluid pressure records are taken with the neck in flexion/extension; if the pressure wave is high this suggests a good deal of instability, impending cord impingement and is an operative indication.

(5) X-rays in flexion and extension are taken: a shift of the odontoid of more than 3 mm ($\frac{1}{8}$ inch) suggests instability (figure 8.1).

(6) Proximal subluxation of the dens as a result of destruction of the occipito-atlanto-axial joints is measured from McGregor's (1948) line which is drawn from the upper surface of the posterior edge of the hard palate to the most caudal point on the occipital curve. If the tip of the odontoid is more than 4.5 mm ($\frac{3}{16}$ inch) above this base line, subluxation is significant.

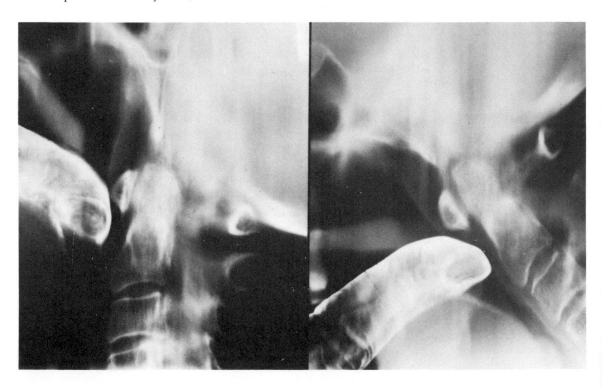

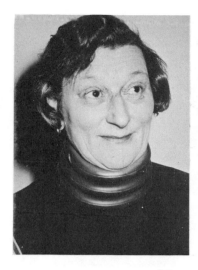
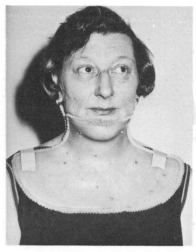
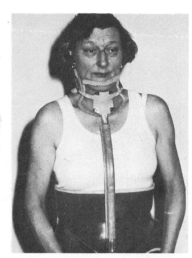

Figure 8.3 Collars of varying grades of rigidity

Treatment

In the presence of symptoms, collar supports providing an increasing degree of rigidity are tried (figure 8.3). If necessary traction in neutral or slight extension relieves symptoms and generally prevents further damage to the cord (figure 8.4). As maintenance of general mobility is vital in rheumatoid disease, a useful method of providing continuous traction is the halopelvic splint (figure

Figure 8.4 Arrangements for (a) temporary neck traction and (b) prolonged neck traction: (a) sling support for traction on the head; (b) skull traction using Blackburn's apparatus

8.5). This consists of a pair of pins which transfix the ilium and a skull caliper; these are connected by bars of variable length. Care must be taken with this device, since considerable traction can be applied without significant discomfort. Also, rapid decalcification of the spine, which occurs with the elimination of gravity produced by the distraction, means that such a splint should be worn for a few weeks only and be applied immediately prior to surgery.

Surgical fusion is indicated when conservative methods fail to control the symptoms and signs of cord compression. A local atlanto-axial interspinous fusion with an H graft of iliac cancellous bone, wired into place, suffices (figures 8.6, 8.14; Simmons and Fielding, 1967). A technical point of

a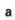

b

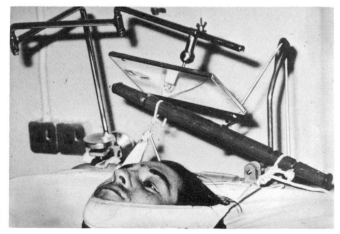
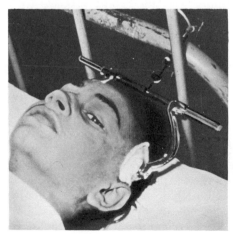

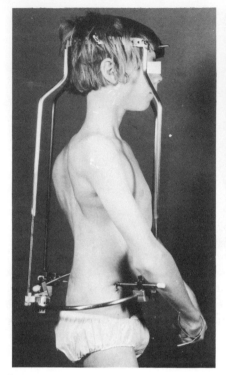

a

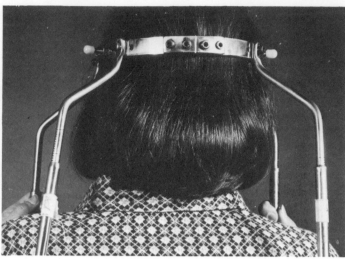

b

Figure 8.5 Halopelvic traction. Note the spring loading on (b)

value is that bone decortication is unnecessary for the graft to fuse, for simple removal of periosteum suffices; bone stock already deficient, is therefore preserved. Anterior local fusion of these vertebrae has to be performed through the pharynx, and grafts so inserted have been expectorated or swallowed: somewhat disconcerting for patient and surgeon alike! Occasionally this is the only route available in the presence of gross bone destruction, but it is not advocated for routine use. An alternative method recently described involves a bilateral approach to the lateral masses necessitating excision of the mastoids. The graft is placed between the lateral masses of atlas and axis (Pahle, 1976).

Atlanto-occipital fusion (Hamblen, 1967; figure 8.7) has a place if the arch of the atlas is flimsy, in failed local intervertebral fusion and where there has been considerable erosion of the lateral masses of the occiput with intracranial subluxation of the odontoid. In atlanto-occipital fusion, tibial or iliac cancellous bone grafts are slotted into gutters cut in the occiput and wired into the spine of the axis,

the intervening spaces being packed with cancellous bone.

An alternative method has been suggested by Brattstrom and Granholm (1973) (figures 8.8, 8.13) using acrylic cement on one side of the spine and cancellous graft on the other; extended immobilisation is then unnecessary and a high fusion rate is reported.

Vertebral collapse, subluxation or dislocation at lower cervical levels is brought about by disc and bone erosion and by pannus from the neurocentral joints. In bone collapse, attempts to effect reduction are usually unsuccessful. If, however, a collar relieves symptoms, then it should be persisted with, for spontaneous fusion and stabilisation can occur. At lower levels in the neck anterior interbody fusion is performed (figures 8.9 and 8.15). In cases with persistent neurological involvement, a posterior decompression should be carried out. Rarely, the denticulate ligaments of the cord have to be divided to allow it to ride posteriorly away from multiple large osteophytes.

Vertebral collapse can also be brought about by mild trauma; corticosteroids may be a contributory or aggravating factor in the porosis leading to such collapse.

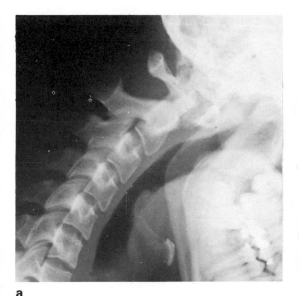

a

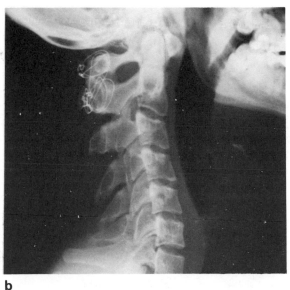

b

Figure 8.6 Atlanto-axial interspinous fusion with H graft wired into place: (a) before, (b) after operation

THE DORSAL AND LUMBAR SPINES

Symptoms at these levels may be due to synovitis of the facetal joints or may arise from damage to vertebral bodies. Osteoporosis resulting from rheumatoid disease is aggravated by immobility, and possibly by corticosteroid therapy, allowing disc intrusion into the softened vertebral bodies, with wedge collapse of the bodies. It is seldom necessary to offer more than a suitable corset support. Occasionally anabolic steroids and supplementary calcium help produce symptomatic relief. Surgical intervention at dorsal or lumbar level is rarely indicated.

THE SPINE IN ANKYLOSING SPONDYLITIS

The diagnosis of ankylosing spondylitis can be difficult. The majority of people with this disease carry HLA B27 antigen, which may be a helpful pointer. Properly supervised patients with ankylosing spondylitis do not develop spinal defor-

Figure 8.7 Occipitocervical fusion

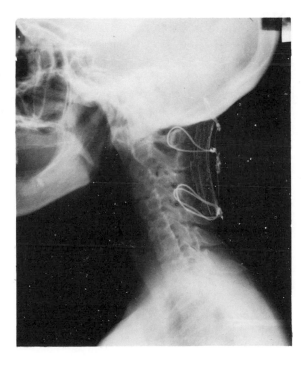

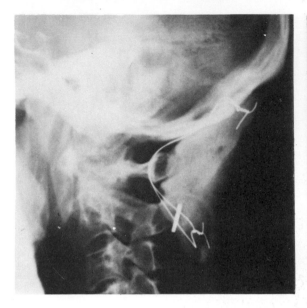

Figure 8.8 Occipitocervical fusion with combined cement and bone graft (H. Brattström)

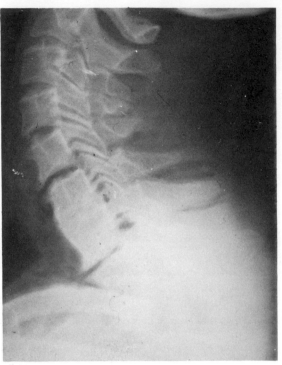

Figure 8.9 Anterior fusion of C6,7

mities, although ankylosis is often inevitable. Adequate medication with, for example, Butazolidin and vigorous exercises may keep patients pain-free and the spine correctly aligned. Splintage is seldom necessary, although Milwaukee braces and more limited forms of bracing can be effective (figure 8.10).

Patients may present with acutely flexed ankylosed spines of such severity as to hamper forward vision; they should be offered surgical correction. Since correction means re-ankylosis in an optimum position, the patient's work and other needs must be considered. Overcorrection may prevent a desk-worker from seeing to write, so that the optimum position has to be carefully assessed. Sight-line photographs are a valuable way of assessing the situation (figure 8.11). It is important to remember that atlanto-axial instability can occur in the presence of a rigid spine and may need surgical stabilisation. Fractures may present in two ways, by slow flexion or sudden flexion; both carry high risks of cord damage. In either case the head tends to droop forwards into a chin-on-chest position; skull traction correction is the method of choice. Halopelvic traction is a most useful device, enabling gradual correction followed by a fusion. In advancing dorsal kyphosis, such traction can

effectively correct deformity and permit Harrington rods to be inserted while bone grafts are added to produce fusion in the corrected position.

Correction of fixed flexion is by classical osteotomy, although more recently, resection osteotomy has been advised; these procedures can be carried out at lower cervical or midlumbar levels. Two forms of osteotomy have been described at lumbar level, one of which is well tried and was originally described by Smith-Petersen, Larson and Aufranc (1945). Law (1959), who has had unparalleled experience of this, reported on 100 unselected cases, many markedly disabled; there was an overall mortality of 8 per cent and correction was well maintained (figure 8.12). Secondly, Goel (1968) described a 'V'-shaped osteotomy between the articular processes with removal of a wedge of bone; he carried this out on 15 patients whom he followed up for 6 years and reported no mortality nor serious complication.

A safe technique is to employ a special brace which will control gradual correction over several days.

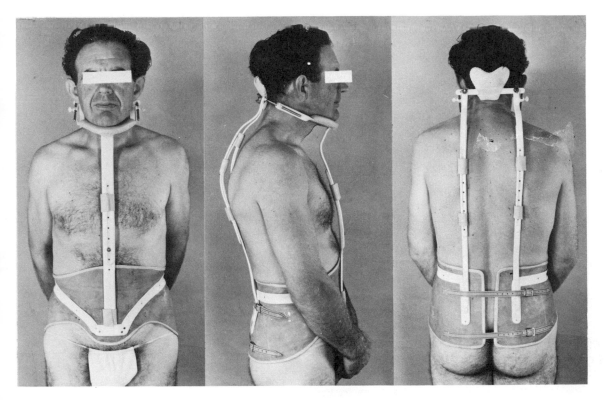

Figure 8.10 The Milwaukee brace

Figure 8.11 Sight line photographs

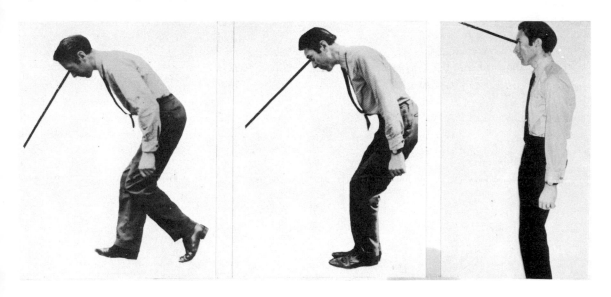

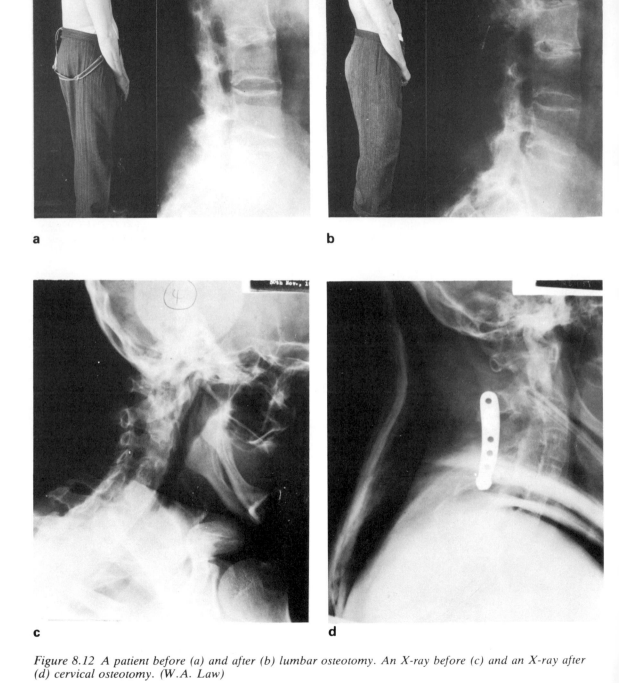

a

b

c

d

Figure 8.12 A patient before (a) and after (b) lumbar osteotomy. An X-ray before (c) and an X-ray after (d) cervical osteotomy. (W.A. Law)

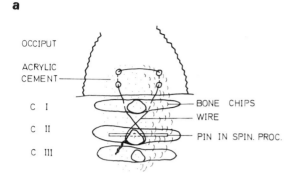

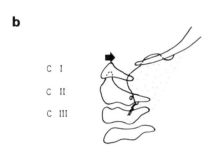

Figure 8.13 Brattström occipitocervical fusion

TECHNIQUES OF OPERATIONS

Occipitocervical fusion (Brattström technique)

The indications are vertical subluxation of the odontoid, failed local atlanto-axial fusion or insufficient bone stock in the atlas to allow a local atlanto-axial fusion. With the patient prone and skull traction applied, a midline incision is made, the suboccipital muscles are separated to expose the occiput and the posterior arches of atlas and axis. Four holes are drilled in the occiput and a Kirschner wire passed transversely through the spinous process of the axis. The exposed bone of one half of the area is rawed. A wire is passed through the holes and lies within the skull on either side of the midline and is on the skull surface where it crosses the midline. Caudally, the wire passes deep to the arch of the atlas and is anchored around the spine of the axis and the transverse pin. The wire is tied and the rawed

area packed with cancellous bone taken from the iliac crest. The other paravertebral gutter is packed with acrylic cement, providing firm and immediate anchorage; keying for the cement is the wire, the small occipital holes and the transverse pin. No external support is necessary (figures 8.8, 8.13).

Gallie's atlanto-axial fusion

The patient is prone and when instability is severe skull traction is applied, a midline incision is made in the suboccipital region; and the muscles are separated to expose the posterior arch of the atlas and the spine of the axis. The periosteum of the exposed laminae of both vertebrae is stripped off. A wire loop is passed under the arch of the atlas and distally around the spine of the axis (figure 8.14). Chips of cancellous bone or an H graft taken from the iliac crest are laid across the rawed areas and between them. The muscles are sutured back and the skin closed. A protective collar with occipital extension is worn for 12 weeks.

Anterior interbody fusion

This is carried out with the patient supine and the head turned away from the side of the incision. Two levels are usual for this operation: at the upper border of the thyroid cartilage, for 2nd to 4th cervical vertebra, and at the lower level of the thyroid cartilage, for 5th to 7th vertebra. X-ray control with markers is mandatory. A transverse skin crease incision is made. Although the recurrent laryngeal nerve is more at risk on the right, it can be identified and protected. On the left the thoracic duct is difficult to find and the consequence of damage more serious. Our preference is for the right-hand side. The platysma is incised vertically and the space between the sternomastoid, laterally and the strap muscles, medially is developed. The carotid sheath is taken laterally and the thyroid medially. The thyroid vessels are divided between ligatures and the prevertebral space entered. The prevertebral fascia is divided to expose the disc space. The correct intervertebral space or spaces are identified and a block of bone cut out. The disc material and vertebral plates are removed, care being taken posteriorly not to

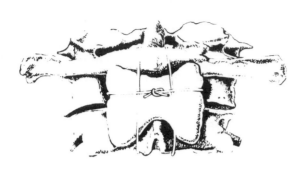

a

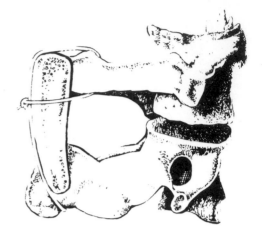

b

Figure 8.14 Technique of wiring in the graft in a Gallie fusion: (a) posterior view; (b) lateral view; (c) X-ray post-operatively

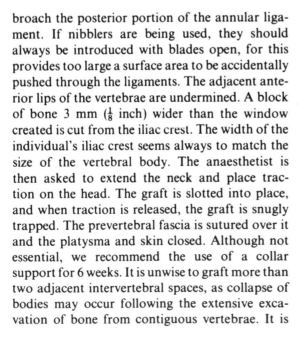

c

broach the posterior portion of the annular ligament. If nibblers are being used, they should always be introduced with blades open, for this provides too large a surface area to be accidentally pushed through the ligaments. The adjacent anterior lips of the vertebrae are undermined. A block of bone 3 mm ($\frac{1}{8}$ inch) wider than the window created is cut from the iliac crest. The width of the individual's iliac crest seems always to match the size of the vertebral body. The anaesthetist is then asked to extend the neck and place traction on the head. The graft is slotted into place, and when traction is released, the graft is snugly trapped. The prevertebral fascia is sutured over it and the platysma and skin closed. Although not essential, we recommend the use of a collar support for 6 weeks. It is unwise to graft more than two adjacent intervertebral spaces, as collapse of bodies may occur following the extensive excavation of bone from contiguous vertebrae. It is

unwise to attempt removal of posterior interbody osteophytes; after fusion these will regress spontaneously (figure 8.15).

Inter-transverse fusion

This can be used at any level but is most commonly employed in the lower lumbar region. The transverse processes are at the axes of vertebral movement in flexion/extension and shift relatively little, in relation to each other, in any one space. The area is sandwiched between vascular muscle bellies and so graft survival and incorporation is rapid, ensuring a high success with only a few days' recumbency necessary post-operatively.

If the spinal canal needs to be explored, a midline incision is used; otherwise it is technically easier to perform the procedure through a transverse skin and muscle cutting incision in the appropriate space. Cancellous graft is taken from the iliac crest and the transverse processes and lateral gutters are rawed. At the lumbosacral interspace the superior aspects of the sacral alae are also rawed. The cancellous grafts are applied and the muscles, deep fascia and skin are closed. The patient may get up when the skin is healed and wears a surgical corset support until fusion is sound; this is usually in 10 weeks.

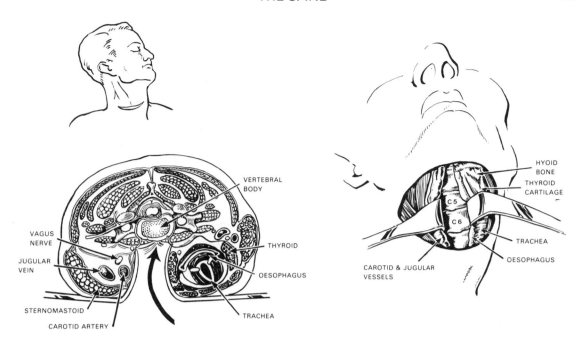

Figure 8.15 Anterior interbody fusion

Skull traction

Three types of apparatus are available: Crutchfield's, Cones' and Blackburn's (figure 8.16). The first two are easier to apply but can accidentally pull out more easily than the last. Cones' prongs are more stable, as they are per-pendicular to the skull and the line of pull, unlike Crutchfield's, which are oblique to both. Blackburn's are preferred, for they fit over the widest portion of the parietal area and the prongs allow firm compression against the inner table of the skull, having an adjustable guard. A guarded drill is used for the holes in the outer table. It is important that this be sharp.

Figure 8.16 Skull calipers: (a) Blackburn skull traction apparatus; (b) Crutchfield skull traction tongs; (c) Stratford modification of Cone ice tong calipers

a   **b**   **c**

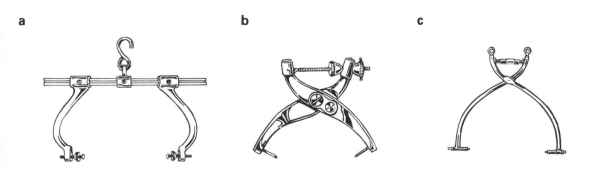

REFERENCES

Brattström, H. and Granholm, L. (1973). Chirurgie der halswirbelsäule bei patienten mit rheumatoider arthritis. *Orthopäde*, **2**, 118–120

Goel, M. K. (1968). Vertebral osteotomy for correction of fixed flexion deformity of the spine. *J. Bone Jt Surg.*, **50A**, 287

Hamblen, D. L. (1967). Occipito-cervical fusion. *J. Bone Jt Surg.*, **49B**, 33

Law, W. A. (1969). Lumbar spine osteotomy. *J. Bone Jt Surg.*, **41B**, 270

McGregor, M. (1948). The significance of certain measurements of the skull in the diagnosis of basilar impression, *Br. J. Radiol.*, **21**, 171

Matthews, J. (1969). Atlanto-axial subluxation in rheumatoid arthritis. *Ann. Rheum. Dis.*, **28**, 260

Pahle, J. (1976). Personal communication

Rana, N. A., Hancock, D. O., Taylor, A. R. and Hill, A. C. S. (1973). 1. Atlanto-axial subluxation in rheumatoid arthritis. 2. Upward translocation of the dens in rheumatoid arthritis. *J. Bone Jt Surg.*, **55B**, 458–477

Simmons, E. H. and Fielding, J. W. (1967). Atlanto-axial arthrodesis by the Gallie technique. *J. Bone Jt Surg.*, **49A**, 1022

Smith-Petersen, M. N., Larson, C. G. and Aufranc, O. E. (1945). Osteotomy of the spine for correction of flexion deformity in rheumatoid arthritis. *J. Bone Jt Surg.*, **27**, 1

9

THE SHOULDER

Movements of the 'shoulder' are complex. These include not only glenohumeral but also scapulo-thoracic motion, which in turn involves both the acromioclavicular and sternoclavicular joints. Thus, when the shoulder joint is the site of complaint, it is essential to examine all these areas.

The early pain of the rheumatoid shoulder may be difficult to distinguish from common, non-rheumatoid conditions such as supraspinatus tendinitis and biceps tendinitis, and the onset is often insidious, stiffness being recognised only when it is too late. The painful shoulder is held in the most comfortable position, often adduction and internal rotation; should fixed deformity occur in this position, considerable loss of function follows. At all times a careful watch is kept for the onset of such deformities and every effort made to prevent them by gentle positioning of the shoulder into abduction and external rotation several times every day, and at night, by resting the upper limb on a pillow. Exercise in a physiotherapy department which includes the use of pulleys may well harm the inflamed tissues and manipulation under an anaesthetic, although tempting when there is limitation of movement, is more likely to do harm than good.

EXTRA-ARTICULAR SOFT TISSUE DISEASE

Subacromial pain

Subacromial pain is common and may be due to subacromial bursitis, supraspinatus tendinitis or degeneration presenting as a painful-arc synd-rome. These conditions may or may not be the result of the rheumatoid disease. Many patients respond to subacromial infiltration of local anaes-thetic, steroid and hyalase and a short period of rest in an arm-sling. Instant and dramatic relief of pain indicates correct placing of the local anaes-thetic; hence the steroid. If relief is not achieved, it is better to repeat the injection immediately.

Severe subacromial pain may be due to de-position of calcium pyrophosphate in the supra-spinatus tendon (figure 9.1). When the pain is acute, the deposit has the consistency of tooth-paste and is under tension. The release of this tension by needling produces immediate relief of pain. Two wide-bore needles may be used and the area washed out with 20 ml of normal saline. Before removing the needles, local anaesthetic and steroid are injected. Positioning of the needles is helped by using an image-intensifier. If a chronic painful-arc syndrome develops and does not respond to local steroid; then a subacromial injection of 8–10 ml of 100 000 centistoke (cS) silicone relieves all but 2 per cent who are resistant to conservative treatment and require surgery.

Surgery is directed towards increasing the subacromial space.

(1) Acromionectomy. This is not recommended, as it weakens the deltoid muscle and frequently does not relieve pain.

(2) Stamm (1963) osteotomy. An osteotomy of the neck of the scapula is made parallel to the plane of the glenoid and 6 mm ($\frac{1}{4}$ inch) from the joint through a posterior incision. The glenoid is then displaced inferiorly to increase the subacromial space. This displacement is not always obvious on X-ray and success may be due sometimes to an unrecognised effect of osteotomy rather than to actual displacement. The arm is rested in a collar and cuff support for 3 weeks and convalescence is rapid.

(3) Neer (1972) anterior acromioplasty. The anterior extremity of the acromion is removed, leaving the attachment of the lateral fibres of the deltoid intact. This anterior acromionectomy thus does little harm but is frequently not associated with pain relief.

(4) Kessel and Watson (1977) recommend excision of the outer end of the clavicle and division of the coraco-acromial ligament for the painful-arc syndrome.

(5) Excision of subacromial bursa. Occasionally there is enormous enlargement of the subacromial bursa. This is excised through an anterior incision, immediately lateral and parallel to the medial border of the deltoid muscle.

Rotator cuff tears

These are not as frequent in rheumatoid disease as is commonly thought. They may be preceded by tendinitis and tendon degeneration. The differentiation between tears and tendinitis is difficult but not important, as the poor collagen tissue makes surgical repair inadvisable. The treatment is as for the painful-arc syndrome unless the elevated hum-

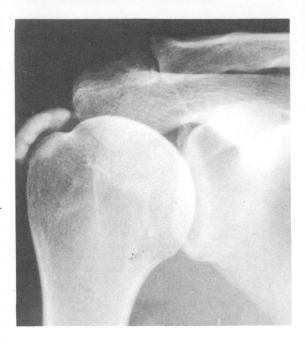

Figure 9.1 Calcium pyrophosphate in the supraspinatus tendon (G. Arden)

eral head requires surgical stabilisation (vide infra).

Bicipital tendinitis

Here pain and tenderness in the region of the bicipital groove is aggravated by supinating and flexing the elbow against resistance. It will usually respond to a short period of rest in an arm-sling and an injection of local anaesthetic, steroid and hyalase. The earlier this injection is given the better is the chance of success. On rare occasions it does not respond to conservative measures and the pain is then almost invariably relieved by excision of the biceps tendon within the bicipital groove and re-insertion by suture of the distal tendon to the periosteum.

Rupture of the long head of the biceps

The diagnosis is obvious, as the muscle bunches when it contracts. No treatment is necessary; in fact, the rupture sometimes results in spontaneous relief of bicipital tendinitis.

Pericapsulitis, frozen shoulder

This syndrome, of shoulder pain, often severe at night and worse during certain arcs of movement, occurs in patients with and without rheumatoid diseases. There is little evidence to support the contention that inflammation is the cause, although inflammatory tissue is usually present in patients with rheumatoid disease. In the non-rheumatoid patient this is usually a self-limiting condition which resolves, often without disability, within 18 months. When rheumatoid disease is the cause of pericapsulitis, pathological changes are evident in both soft tissues and bone, and the subsequent disability is due to these changes. Non-rheumatoid pericapsulitis can cause almost complete immobility of the shoulder, unassociated with observable pathological changes; fortunately full movement usually returns spontaneously. Probably a similar process occurs in the rheumatoid patient but the prolonged immobility results in permanent stiffness due to the superimposed rheumatoid pathology. Whereas it is helpful to use the terms 'supraspinatus tendinitis' and 'bicipital tendinitis', these conditions are frequently part of a general pericapsulitis. The most disagreeable aspect of pericapsulitis is night pain; usually this responds to a short rest period in a sling and an injection of local anaesthetic, steroid and hyalase into the most painful area.

Periscapular pain

Infrascapular fasciitis and subscapular rheumatoid bursitis often respond to simple rest and heat. When a tender nodule is palpable, an injection of local anaesthetic, steroid and hyalase is frequently effective; the injection is directed towards a rib to reduce the chance of pleural puncture.

Suprascapular nerve compression

Pain experienced at the apex of the shoulder and in the suprascapular fossa may be relieved by local anaesthetic injection or by decompression of the suprascapular nerve, in the suprascapular notch medial to the base of the coracoid process.

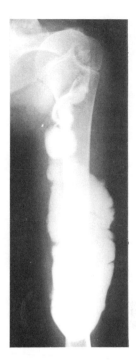

Figure 9.2 Synovial cyst. Arthrogram of shoulder. (G. Arden)

Synovial cysts

These may extend as far as the elbow (figure 9.2) and require excision.

INTRA-ARTICULAR DISEASE

The acromioclavicular joint

When this joint is damaged by rheumatoid synovitis and erosions (figure 9.3), the resulting pain appears to arise in the glenohumeral joint. Careful examination will reveal tenderness localised to the acromioclavicular joint, which, infiltrated with local anaesthetic, temporarily relieves the pain and tenderness, while steroid injections produce lasting relief. Rarely, when conservative measures fail, resection of the lateral end of the clavicle is indicated.

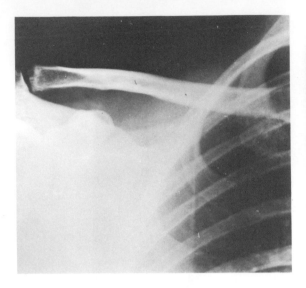 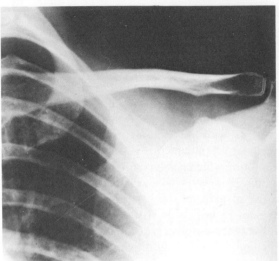

Figure 9.3 This patient presented with shoulder pain which was completely relieved following an injection into the diseased right acromioclavicular joint

The sternoclavicular joint

This joint may also be affected by synovitis and erosions and may sublux, but is less frequently the site of pain than the acromioclavicular joint; steroid injections usually give relief. The indications for surgery are rare; synovectomy and débridement is preferable to excision of the medial end of the clavicle.

The glenohumeral joint

Pain from this joint is referred to the humeral insertion of the deltoid muscle. It is essential to realise that all glenohumeral movements are combined with those of the acromioclavicular, sternoclavicular and scapulothoracic articulations. Shoulder abduction is a co-ordinated movement of the humerus, the scapula and the clavicle. Normally all three move together, some scapulothoracic movement occurring immediately after the initiation of abduction.

Synovitis

This is characterised by swelling and pain on movement, usually relieved by rest and a local injection of steroid.

Pyarthrosis

Sepsis in the rheumatoid shoulder, as in other rheumatoid joints, is easily misdiagnosed. It should always be considered in the presence of a recent therapeutic injection.

Subluxation of the head of the humerus

Subluxation is generally superior (figure 9.4a), and is probably related to deltoid spasm which splints the glenohumeral joint during movement at the scapulothoracic joint. It may be associated with inhibition of the supraspinatus muscle, which thus fails to anchor the head of the humerus at its correct level with the glenoid. Less commonly there may be a tear or stretching of the rotator cuff. Pain can inhibit the deltoid muscle, causing inferior subluxation of the humeral head, which recovers when the pain resolves (figure 9.4b).

Treatment

Treatment of the glenohumeral subluxation may be conservative, by physiotherapy directed to increasing abduction and rotation by Menell manipulations in which the joint is moved while applying continuous traction to the arm (chapter 1), or by operative treatment. The latter includes silicone rubber interposition or pectoralis minor transplant.

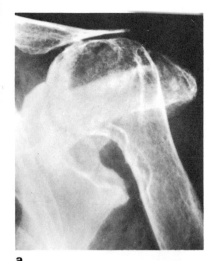 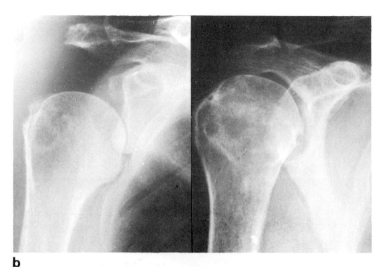

a   b

Figure 9.4 (a) Synovitis here has eroded the medial aspect of the humeral neck and has stretched the supraspinatus tendon allowing upward subluxation of the humeral head. An arthrogram did not reveal a capsular tear; (b) inferior subluxation of the humeral head in a painful shoulder; 3 weeks later elevation of the shoulder to its normal position after relief of pain by medical treatment

Silicone rubber interposition The insertion of a subacromial silastic block, made of soft-grade silicone 'rubber,' has improved function for 2 years. This block, theoretically, holds the head of the humerus down, giving the deltoid a mechanical advantage when abducting the arm.

Pectoralis minor transplant Transplantation of the pectoralis minor insertion from the medial border of the coracoid process to the great tuberosity of the humerus enables it to act directly upon the head of the humerus, thus stabilising it. This reverts the muscle to its early phylogenetic function and mimics that still found in birds, stabilising the shoulder on the down-beat of wing motion. The pectoralis minor was originally inserted into the head of the humerus; during evolution the coracoid process insinuated its way into the tendon and the coracohumeral ligament is the remnant of the tendon and its humeral attachment.

This operation was first performed (Helal, 1977) on a Scottish international rugby player who did not have rheumatoid arthritis and whose supra-

spinatus tendon had been twice repaired unsuccessfully.

The operative technique is simple: the insertion is transferred with a sliver of coracoid bone to the supraspinatus facet on the head of the humerus, a distance of 2 cm ($\sim \frac{3}{4}$ inch) and held there with a staple.

The indication in rheumatoid disease is a shoulder with superior subluxation of the humerus which cannot be actively abducted but can be elevated after traction on the arm and stabilisation of the head of the humerus by the examining hand (figure 9.5).

The upwardly subluxed head of the humerus also resumes a more correct relation with the glenoid, following a successful shoulder double osteotomy (figure 9.7).

Severe rheumatoid changes in the articular surfaces

The indications for surgery depend almost entirely on pain and to a lesser extent on loss of function. The treatment is conservative initially; deep heat and a short period of rest or an injection of hydrocortisone may give lasting relief despite gross radiological changes in the joint. Severe bony damage is compatible with many years of freedom from pain and little loss of function. Only when these changes are associated with persistent pain, uncontrolled by simple measures, is surgery justified.

Figure 9.5 (a) Active abduction impossible owing to supraspinatus inaction: (b) full active abduction after the humeral head had been stabilised by the examining hand

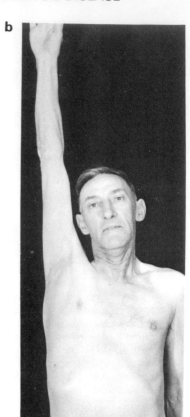

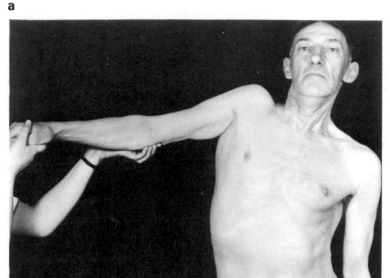

Synovectomy

If there is significant swelling of the shoulder joint, synovectomy may prove beneficial. Through an anterior incision as much of the synovium as can be reached is excised. Post-operatively the shoulder is immobilised in a few degrees of abduction and flexion for only 1 week. This operation has been described in association with various soft tissue procedures intended to release the adhesions and contractures which hold the diseased joint in adduction and internal rotation. Such an operation seldom results in a significant increase in movement and is not advised.

Double Osteotomy

Severe shoulder pain of many years' duration may be alleviated by this simple but effective operation (Benjamin, 1974). While glenohumeral movement including rotation is retained, it is never increased, whereas the range of total 'shoulder' movement is considerably increased. Between 1967 and 1975, 16 patients with severe shoulder pain, restricted movements, loss of upper limb function and well-marked radiographic changes were treated by double osteotomy. Twelve of the sixteen patients suffered from rheumatoid disease; They were reviewed in 1976 (Benjamin, Arden and Hirschowitz, 1977).

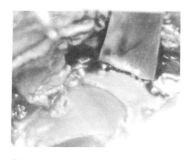
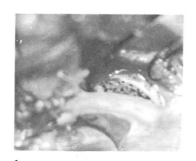
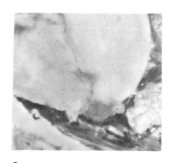

a   b   c

Figure 9.6 Operative technique for double osteotomy of the shoulder: (a) osteotome about to make the glenoid cut; (b) the glenoid osteotomy; (c) the humeral neck osteotomy

Operative technique

Through an anterior shoulder-strap incision, the fibres of the deltoid muscle are separated parallel to and 12 mm ($\frac{1}{2}$ inch) lateral to the deltopectoral groove; the tip of the coracoid process is detached and the subscapularis muscle divided. Two pairs of bone levers are inserted, one above and below the neck of the glenoid, and the other pair, on either side of the surgical neck of the humerus.

The glenoid osteotomy is performed 5 mm($\sim \frac{1}{4}$ inch) medial to the glenoid fossa and parallel with it; the humeral osteotomy is at the level of the surgical neck. Both are without displacement, osteotomes cutting all but the posterior cortices. The osteotomies are completed when the osteotomes lever open the posterior cortices hinging

Figure 9.7 Double osteotomy of the shoulder: (a) pre-operative—notice the subluxation; (b) 10 days post-operative; (c) 2 years post-operative

the bones on intact posterior periosteum (figures 9.6 and 9.7).

The arm is supported in a sling and active shoulder exercises commenced on the tenth post-operative day.

Results

Movement

The total active range of shoulder abduction was measured pre- and post-operatively (figure 9.8a); in 13 cases this increased by an average of 50°. This improvement in the functional range is probably due to relief of pain and muscle spasm; no example of increased glenohumeral movement was observed. The average post-operative range of rotation was 66°.

Pain

Thirteen of the sixteen patients post-operatively had either no pain or slight occasional pain. Two were improved, with slight residual pain, and one was not improved (figure 9.8b).

a   b   c

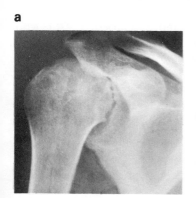
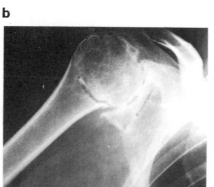
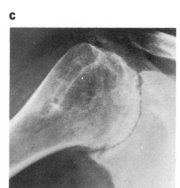

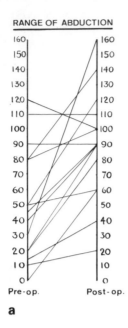

a

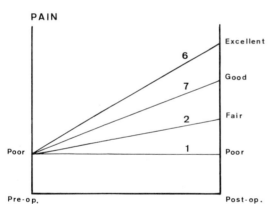

b

Figure 9.8 Double osteotomy results, 16 cases: (a) total active range of shoulder abduction. The post-operative increase is largely due to scapulothoracic mobility; (b) pain relief

Function

Functional improvement was directly related to pain relief. For example, two patients with severe rheumatoid disease who had been unable to use crutches were able to do so following double osteotomy.

Complications

There were no serious complications. Non-union of the humeral osteotomy with ankylosis of the glenohumeral joint occurred in one patient. She had 90° of abduction and 80° of rotation with virtually no pain 2 years after operation.

Case report

J.B. was 25 years of age in 1967 and suffered from rheumatoid disease with a slide latex titre of 1246. Incapacitating pain in the shoulder severely limited upper limb function and sleep was disturbed for 2 years. The pain failed to respond to medical treatment, including systemic steroid therapy. Radiographs revealed severe rheumatoid disease of the shoulder; she was referred to the orthopaedic department for arthrodesis but became the first patient to undergo double osteotomy of the shoulder. By error the glenoid osteotomy was incomplete, breaking into the articular surface. There could thus have been no inferior displacement of the glenoid (figure 9.9a). Two weeks after operation her pain was entirely relieved and total shoulder abduction was 90°. During the subsequent 7 years she married, brought up two children and remained entirely pain-free (figure 9.10). The recent radiographs show that the previously elevated humeral head has descended to its correct position and the joint space and bony structure appear to have improved (figure 9.9b).

GLENOIDECTOMY

Excision of the glenoid has been described by Wainwright (1974) and by Gariepy (1976), who claim that it relieves pain with little interference with function.

EXCISION OF THE HEAD OF THE HUMERUS

This procedure, which destroys the fulcrum of the shoulder and interferes severely with function, is not recommended.

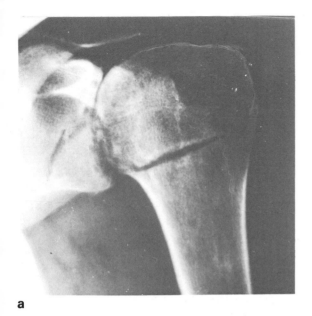

a

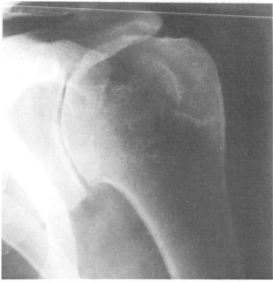

b

Figure 9.9 The first shoulder double osteotomy: (a) 1967—the glenoid cut was unintentionally incomplete; (b) 1976—entirely pain-free

Figure 9.10 Nine years after shoulder osteotomy for incapacitating pain

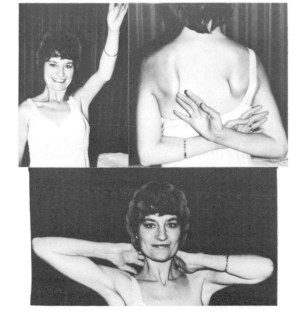

ARTHRODESIS

Arthrodesis is technically difficult and involves cumbersome post-operative immobilisation. If successful, glenohumeral pain is relieved, but the consequent loss of movement, particularly of glenohumeral rotation, reduces function and throws increased stress on other upper limb joints. Internal fixation by a compression screw is considered the best method if arthrodesis is indicated.

HEMI-JOINT REPLACEMENT

The insertion of a prosthetic humeral head is not recommended, as the diseased glenoid is inadequate to articulate with the prosthesis (figure 9.11).

TOTAL JOINT REPLACEMENT

No satisfactory prosthetic shoulder replacement has yet been developed. The shoulder depends for its stability and function on muscles and tendons—in particular, the rotator cuff which anchors the head of the humerus to the glenoid

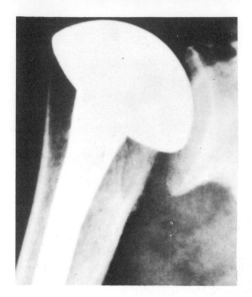

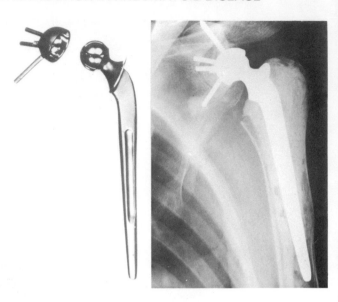

Figure 9.11 The Neer prosthesis

Figure 9.12 The Stanmore shoulder (A. Lettin and Institute of Orthopaedics)

during abduction. Failure to increase the range of active glenohumeral abduction following replacement is due to the absence of a functioning rotator cuff. Rheumatoid disease invades the rotator cuff and prevents its satisfactory reconstruction.

Owing to the small bulk of the scapula, fixation of the prosthesis requires ingenuity of design which is still not perfected. Some prostheses mimic the anatomical arrangement (figure 9.12), whereas others employ the reversed ball-and-socket principle (figure 9.13), in which the ball is the proximal component and the socket is distal. By this means scapular fixation is said to be improved.

Laurence is experimenting with a shoulder similar in design to a hip prosthesis. The cup is positioned beneath the acromion and coracoid and is intended to stabilise the head, thus enabling shoulder abduction without the rotator cuff (figure 9.14).

A shoulder prosthesis may be slightly constrained where stability relies on its configuration associated with soft tissue support; it may be totally constrained, as in the self-retained reverse ball-and-socket (Ranawat and Poppen, 1977); or partially constrained, in which the inherent stability is limited, allowing dislocation under traumatic loading with the prospect of closed reduction (Beddow and Elloy, 1977).

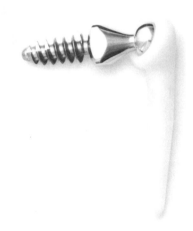

Figure 9.13 The Kessel shoulder. The metal ball component is inserted into the scapula and the plastic socket into the humerus (L. Kessel and Institute of Orthopaedics)

The objectives so far achieved by the shoulder prostheses are limited. Pain relief with no loss and little, if any, gain in mobility is all that is claimed.

The potential complications of total shoulder replacements are considerable, and similar results at present are achieved by double osteotomy, which is simple, free from complications and

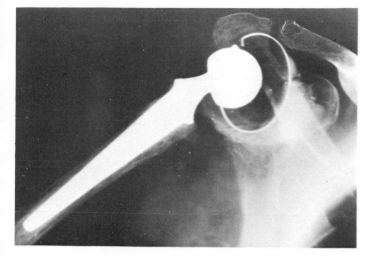 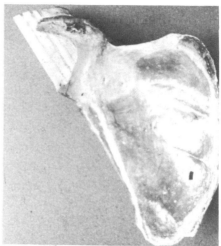

Figure 9.14 The Laurence shoulder. The large cup fits below the acromion and coracoid processes (M. Laurence)

allows further surgery to the shoulder, including prosthetic replacement if pain is not relieved.

CRUTCHES

The use of crutches in rheumatoid disease of the lower limb throws undue strain upon the upper limb joints, which are not designed for bearing the entire body-weight. Nevertheless, if crutches are necessary, it is better to avoid axillary crutches, as these throw particular strain on the shoulders. Elbow crutches with forearm gutters distribute weight along the length of the forearm and diminish it in the hand; thus reducing the danger of damage to the distal upper limb joints.

CONCLUSION

The upper limb is a single functional unit and it is to be remembered that the shoulder joint is entirely subservient to the needs of the hand. If the hand is able to be placed without undue pain according to the requirements of the patient, then the function of the shoulder is adequate. So long as the patient is able to comb hair without undue pain, deal with dress and sleep, satisfaction is likely and treatment to regain more shoulder movement is meddlesome and undesirable.

REFERENCES

Beddow, F. H. and Elloy, M. A. (1977). The Liverpool total replacement for the gleno-humeral joint. *Conference on Joint Replacement in the Upper Limb* (abstracts), Mechanical Engineering Publications, London

Benjamin, A. (1974). Double osteotomy of the shoulder. *Scand. J. Rheum.*, **3**, 65

Benjamin, A., Arden, G. P. and Hirschowitz, D. (1977). The treatment of arthritis of the shoulder joint by double osteotomy. *Int. Rheum. Meeting*, San Francisco.

Gariepy, R. (1976). Glenoidectomy in the repair of the rheumatoid shoulder. 6th *Combined Meeting Orth. Ass. Eng. Speaking World*, London

Helal, B. (1977). Pectoralis minor transfer. *Br. Orthopaedic Study Group* Zurs

Kessel, L. and Watson, M. (1977). The painful arc syndrome. *J. Bone Jt Surg*, **59B,** 166–172

Laurence, M. (1976). Personal communication

Neer, C. S. (1972). Anterior acromioplasty for the chronic impingement syndrome in the shoulder. *J. Bone Jt Surg*, **54A,** 41–50

Ranawat, C. S. and Poppen, N. (1977). Total shoulder prosthesis. *Conference on Joint Replacement in the Upper Limb* (abstracts), Mechanical Engineering Publications, London

Stamm, T. T. (1963). New operation for chronic subcoracoid bursitis. *J. Bone Jt Surg.*, **45B,** 207

Wainwright, D. (1974). Glenoidectomy: A method of treating the painful shoulder in severe rheumatoid arthritis. *Ann. Rheum. Dis.*, **33**(1), 110

10

THE ELBOW

Elbow function, especially in the intermediate range of movement, is important to independence. Events such as eating, dressing and perineal toilet depend upon a certain degree of elbow movement in both flexion/extension and rotation. Stability is also important, for it becomes a weight-bearing joint when crutches are used; thus, in considering surgical priorities, it may be necessary to solve an elbow problem in advance of lower limb surgery to enable the patient to use walking aids.

EXTRA-ARTICULAR DISEASE

Fasciitis

This may be a prodromal symptom of rheumatoid disease. The attacks may occur repetitively and at multiple sites; patients complain of pain in the region of the common flexor muscles origin in 'golfers elbow' or about the common extensor muscles origin in 'tennis elbow'. Their pain is aggravated by use of the hand, particularly when gripping and lifting. These syndromes are also referred to as 'epicondylitis' and in rheumatoid arthritis must be distinguished from the articular pain of synovitis or arthritis and from ulnar neuritis. The tenderness over the respective epicondyles of the humerus, external in 'tennis' elbow and internal in 'golfers' elbow, often responds to an injection of steroid; combined with a local anaesthetic, the immediate relief of pain is then an indication that the steroid has been correctly placed. A session of ultrasonic treatment immediately following steroid injection seems to enhance the effect. Resistant cases are usually those of 'tennis' elbow, for which a number of aetiological factors have been blamed, and thus treatment varies. It is probable the condition is multifactorial, so examination must be meticulous to identify the precise cause. The majority are due to small tears of the common extensor origin and recurrence is due to re-tearing of the repaired fibrous tissue. Surgical detachment of the origin appears to give rise to no functional disability and will cure the majority of resistant cases. Although the reason is not clear, an elasticated band, compressing the forearm just below the epicondyles, will allow pain-free vigorous use of the hand while the device is being worn.

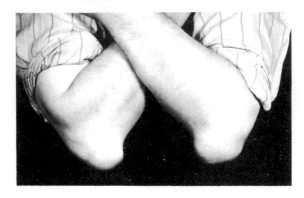

Figure 10.1 Rheumatoid olecranon bursitis

Sixth cervical root irritation will give rise to pain in the same area, and enquiry about and examination of the neck and upper limb, including its neurology, will identify this cause.

A tight extensor carpi radialis brevis as a cause has been propounded by Garden (1961); some patients respond to elongation of this tendon in the lower forearm. Bosworth (1955) believes that stenosis and thickening of the orbicular ligament is a cause; such patients respond to excision of this ligament. In these cases tenderness is over the ligament. Roles and Maudsley (1972) believe that some patients have pain due to entrapment of the posterior interosseous nerve, causing weakness of finger dorsiflexors and electrical evidence of reduced conduction. Newman and Goodfellow (1975) suggest other cases are due to fibrillation of the radial head, which can be identified by pain relief following intra-articular local anaesthesia.

It is clearly important to assess all possibilities before embarking upon surgical measures for resistant 'tennis' elbow.

Tendinitis

Tendinitis of the insertion of the biceps may occur as part of the rheumatoid inflammatory process. Local infiltration with hydrocortisone is effective.

Bursitis

Inflammation of the olecranon bursa is frequent in rheumatoid disease (figure 10.1). It is usually

recurrent or long-standing and is best treated by surgical excision of the bursa. It is prudent to rest the elbow in a plaster back slab until the skin has healed. This bursa may communicate with the joint, and cases of delayed healing after its excision may be due to synovial fistula; should this happen, formal joint synovectomy is the best solution.

Nerve compressions

The ulnar nerve traverses a fibrous tunnel behind the medial epicondyle of the humerus. The bony wall gives way to a capsular wall as the nerve proceeds distally between two heads of the flexor carpi ulnaris. When the joint capsule is distended by synovial thickening or by effusion, the ulnar tunnel is narrowed and symptoms of ulnar nerve irritation may ensue. In its mildest form, paraesthesiae are felt in the ulnar one-and-a-half digits. More severe and persistent compression will give rise to numbness in the same distribution and possibly to weakness of the ulnar intrinsics of the hand, with clawing of the ring and little fingers.

Decompression by incision of the tunnel roof is sometimes sufficient to relieve symptoms (Osborne, 1957). However, more permanent relief will be afforded by anterior transposition of the nerve; this is especially important in a disease which may give rise to fixed flexion and possibly valgus instability of the elbow. On transposition, the nerve may be placed in the subcutaneous tissue or deep to the muscle on bone and joint capsule. In the latter case the common flexor origin is incised or detached from bone and reflected. This deeper repositioning of the nerve gives protection and probably a better blood supply. Operations on the nerve behind the epicondyle are best carried out with the patient prone, for this gives easy access to the medial side of the elbow. It is therefore prudent to check beforehand that the patient can get his arm behind his back, as often the shoulder is concurrently involved in rheumatoid disease.

The posterior interosseous nerve is not infrequently compressed by subluxation or synovitis where it passes anterolaterally at the level of the radial head. The resultant 'dropped' fingers in the rheumatoid hand may be confused with 'attrition' ruptures (chapter 12).

INTRA-ARTICULAR DISEASE

Synovitis

Acute episodes often respond to intra-articular injections of steroid. Chronic synovitis, causing pain and stiffness, is best treated by synovectomy. Chemical synovectomy with Thiotepa, radioactive gold and other materials has given variable results and sometimes causes unwanted damage to the articular cartilage and at worst chemical chondrolysis. Surgical synovectomy is probably less damaging. The radial side of the joint is invariably eroded and radial head excision will facilitate synovectomy (Torgerson and Leach, 1970). The articular cartilage of the radial head was abnormal in 22 such synovectomies carried out in our unit. In the past 5 years we have inserted a silicone rubber radial head in 18 patients, aiming to provide additional stability for the elbow, which sometimes drifts into valgus after head removal. Such elbows function satisfactorily but have yet to be assessed long-term. Synovectomy has produced lasting relief of pain and return of function in 12 of 16 patients reviewed over a 5 year period by Porter, Richardson and Vainio (1974). Wilson, Arden and Ansell (1973) confirm the value of synovectomy. It is important, of course, to preserve the head of the radius in children; otherwise growth imbalance with valgus deformity will occur.

Erosive disease with and without instability

When the joint is unstable, surgical treatment is the best solution; while splintage of the elbow gives relief, it is functionally limiting. In the stable, stiff, grating elbow an intra-articular injection of 8–10 ml of 100 000 cS silicone provides permanent relief in 12 per cent and temporary relief in 88 per cent of patients; it is always worth a trial.

ARTHRODESIS

Arthrodesis with the elbow at a right angle will relieve pain but is a considerable functional handicap and has virtually been abandoned.

ARTHROPLASTY OF THE ELBOW

Excision arthroplasty

Excision arthroplasty or fascial arthroplasty results in an unstable joint in many cases (Knight and Van Landt, 1952).

Before this procedure on the elbow, the ulnar nerve, which is vulnerable behind the medial epicondyle, should be identified, mobilised and transposed anteriorly. Simple excision of the distal humerus and olecranon gives a mobile, painless but unstable elbow (figure 10.2). Alternatively the radial head and the olecranon notch is cleared and the distal humerus excised between the supracondylar ridges, which are then made to fork over the olecranon notch: the so-called 'forked stick' pseudarthrosis (figure 10.3). This may give a surprisingly stable elbow and is the method of choice for salvaging a prosthetic failure.

Fascial or skin arthroplasty

After excising the articular surfaces, the bone-ends are lined with a double layer of fascia lata or of skin. Results are not very predictable; many elbows so treated become weak and unstable, and others stiff owing to excessive fibrosis.

Silicone rubber interposition arthroplasty
(Helal, 1974; figure 10.4)

Through a lateral approach, radial head excision and synovectomy are performed and a 3 mm ($\frac{1}{8}$ inch) thick, curved piece of silastic rubber (silicone rubber spacer manufactured by A. C. Roberts, 3 Rein Road, Morley, Leeds, Yorkshire) is placed in the olecranon notch; the excised radial head is replaced by a Swanson silicone rubber head of radius, if the joint tends to collapse into valgus. Post-operatively, the elbow is protected in a plaster cast at 90° for 2 weeks. Twelve patients, with a follow-up from 2 to 6 years have been assessed; one had the silastic spacer removed following infection and developed a stable pseudarthrosis; none complained of pain; two were unstable; extension lacked 10–15° in eleven; flexion and rotation were full in all.

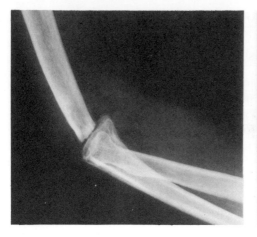
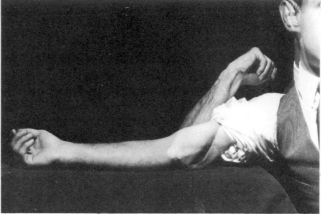

Figure 10.2 An excision arthroplasty. Good 'active' stability and excellent movement

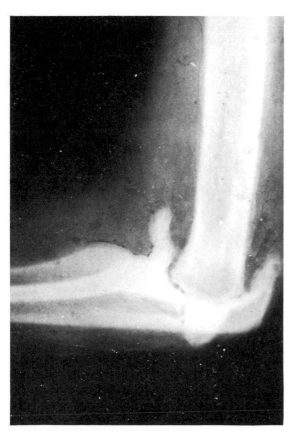

Figure 10.3 The 'forked stick' pseudoarthrosis

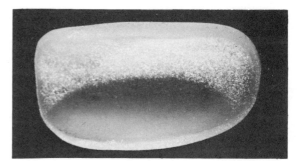

Figure 10.4 Silicone rubber spacer

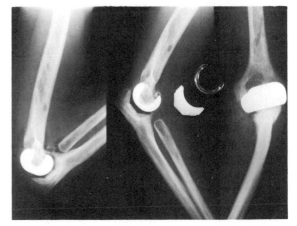

Figure 10.5 ICLH prosthesis (B. Roper and M. Tuke)

Resurfacing prosthesis

Several prostheses have been designed to provide a simple resurfacing of the elbow joint.

The ICLH (Imperial College London Hospital) prosthesis (figure 10.5), developed by Roper *et al.* (London Hospital, 1977) and Tuke, consists of a metal roller which surfaces the trochlea and a polythene concave element which fits the olecranon notch; both are cemented in place. A posterior approach is made; after mobilising and transposing the ulnar nerve the triceps is divided through its aponeurosis. If deformed, the radial head is removed through the same incision. A radial head prosthesis is not necessary, as stability is adequate. The surfaces are shaped with the aid of guides. After 1 year's experience in six elbows, no more than guarded optimism can be expressed.

Lowe and Miller (1977) have described a prosthesis with a metal component in the olecranon notch and polythene on the trochlear surface (figure 10.6); it has been inserted in four patients and the results are considered encouraging.

The prosthesis of Cavendish and Elloy (1977) in Liverpool has a humeral component made of metal, with the desirable design feature that anchorage depends on well-preserved supracondylar ridges. They report two failures in ten cases followed up from 1 to 2½ years.

Humeral resurfacing hemiarthroplasty (Stevens 1977)

From a medial approach this device is keyed to the prepared surface of the lower humerus (figure 10.7). Experience of 18 cases suggests it should not be used in 'bone formers' or haemophiliacs.

Stemmed unconstrained arthroplasty

Ewald (1977) (figure 10.8) has designed a stemmed humeral component articulating with a polythene-resurfaced ulna. Fifty such prostheses have been implanted in 46 patients, with a follow-up ranging from 6 months to 3 years. The four failures followed previous fascial arthroplasty, previous infection and occurred in the presence of severe cubitus valgus.

A stemmed stabilised sliding prosthesis

Attenborough has designed an elbow prosthesis on a similar principle to his knee joint design (figure 10.9). Clinical trials are in an early phase.

Figure 10.6 The Lowe–Miller condylar replacement (L. Lowe)

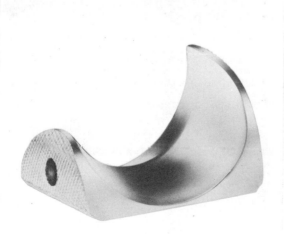
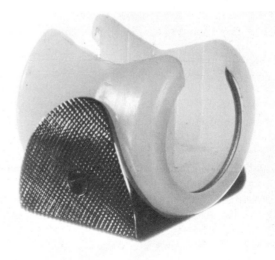

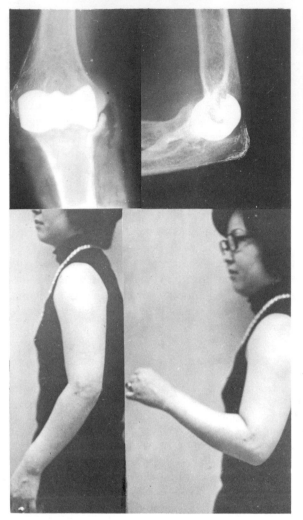

Figure 10.7 The Stevens elbow (P.S. Stevens)

Hinge prostheses

Experience with the Dee (1972) prosthesis (figure 10.10) has been in the main unhappy, principally owing to loosening of the stems (Souter, 1973). In 1977 Dee spoke of its faults and called the prosthesis obsolete: a 7-year cycle from inception to obsolescence. A salutary orthopaedic lesson suggests that careful observation would avoid the imposition of prostheses with bad design faults on the world at large and so confine calamities to a relative few, all under the control of the originator.

Scales and Lettin (1977) have persisted with a prolonged trial of the Stanmore hinge (figure 10.11), which they tested clinically for several years before making it available. This prosthesis has a better stem design than the Dee hinge and fixation has been improved by the use of a cement introducer, essential for inserting cement down the narrow medulla of the ulna. A long follow-up of 8 years or more has revealed few failures.

NOTES ON OPERATIVE TECHNIQUE

Care must be taken to find, mobilise and transpose the ulnar nerve from behind the medial epicondyle, where it is especially vulnerable. The edge of the medial intermuscular septum should be divided to avoid compression of the transposed nerve. The posterior interosseous branch of the radial nerve is also vulnerable, as it courses through the supinator in an anterolateral relationship to the radial head, and care must be taken to avoid stretching by retractors.

In the posterior approach to the elbow, the triceps needs to be reflected, either by cutting the muscle in its aponeurosis or detaching its insertion with a fragment of the olecranon which can be easily screwed back into place.

In applying wool and bandages the elbow is held at a right angle. If the dressings are applied with the elbow straight and subsequently it is flexed to a right angle, then there is danger of circulatory obstruction.

CONCLUSION

A cautious approach to implant arthroplasty is advised: an interposition with silicone rubber is a totally retrievable situation; the surfacing prostheses are a second line of action; the hinge prosthesis is required for the very unstable elbow; and lastly the 'forked stick' type of excision arthroplasty is the final salvage retreat.

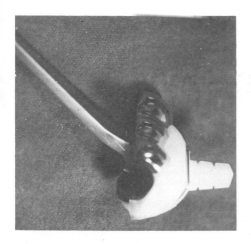

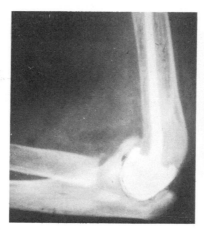

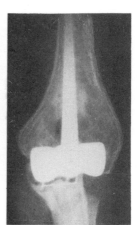

Figure 10.8 The Ewald elbow (F.C. Ewald)

Fig 10.9 The Attenborough elbow (C. Attenborough)

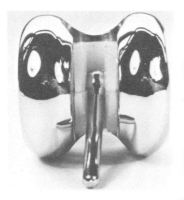

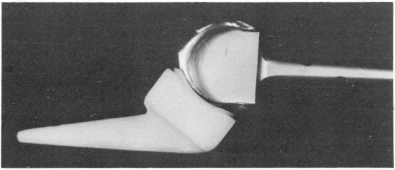

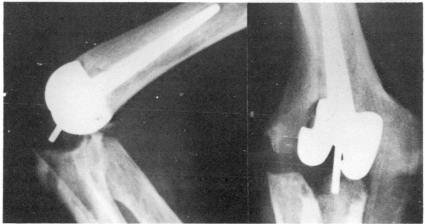

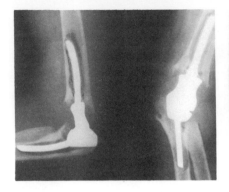

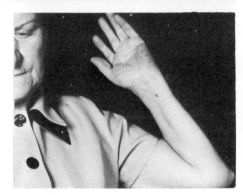

Figure 10.10 Dee hinge arthroplasty. Excellent pain-less movement is preserved 5 years post-operatively, despite X-ray evidence of loose stems

Figure 10.11 Stanmore hinge. Bilateral elbow re-placements (J. Scales)

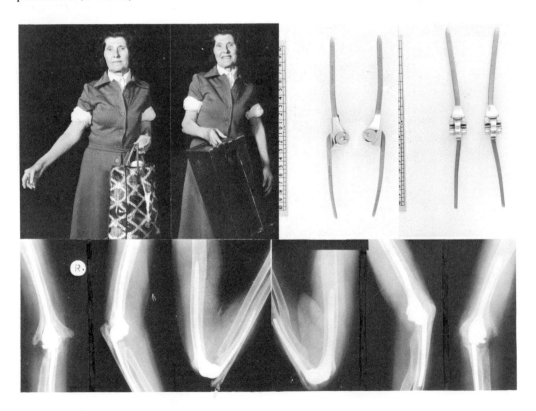

REFERENCES

Bosworth, M. D. (1955). The role of the orbicular ligament in tennis elbow. *J. Bone Jt Surg.*, **37A**, 527–533

Cavendish, M. E. and Elloy, M. A. (1977). A simple method of total elbow replacement. *British Orthopaedic Association Meeting*

Dee, R. (1972). Total replacement arthroplasty of the elbow for rheumatoid arthritis. *J. Bone Jt Surg.*, **54B**, 88

Ewald, F. C., Thomas, W. H., Sledge, C. B., Scott, R. D. and Poss, R. (1977). Non-constrained metal to plastic total elbow arthroplasty in rheumatoid arthritis. *Conference on Joint Replacement of the Upper Limb* (abstracts), Mechanical Engineering Publications Ltd, p. 15

Garden, R. S. (1961). Tennis elbow. *J. Bone Jt Surg.*, **43B**, 100–106

Helal, B. (1974). *Proc. Rheum. Arth. Surg. Soc.* – Norwich Meeting.

Knight, R. A. and Van Landt, I. L. (1952). Arthroplasty of the elbow. *J. Bone Jt Surg.*, **34A**, 610–618

Lowe, L. W. and Miller, A. J. (1977). Condylar replacement of the elbow joint. *Conference on Joint Replacement of the Upper Limb* (abstracts), Mechanical Engineering Publications Ltd, p. 13

Newman, J. H. and Goodfellow, J. W. (1975). Fibrillation of the head of radius, one cause for tennis elbow. *J. Bone Jt Surg.*, **57B**, 15

Osborne, G. V. (1957). Surgical treatment of tardy ulnar neuritis. *J. Bone Jt Surg.*, **39B**, 782

Porter, B. B., Richardson, C. and Vainio, K. (1974). *J. Bone Jt Surg.*, **56B**, No. 3, 427

Roles, N. C. and Maudsley, R. H. (1972). Radial tunnel syndrome. *J. Bone Jt Surg.*, **54B**, 499–508

Roper, B. A. and Swanson, S. A. V. (1977). I.C.L.H elbow prosthesis. *Conference on Joint Replacement of the Upper Limb* (abstracts), Mechanical Engineering Publications Ltd, p. 10

Scales, J. T., Lettin, A. W. F. and Bayley, I. (1977). The evolution of the Stanmore hinged total elbow replacement 1967–76. *Conference on Joint Replacement of the Upper Limb* (abstracts), Mechanical Engineering Publications Ltd, p. 11

Souter, W. A. (1973). Metallic hinge arthroplasty in the elbow joint. *J. Bone Jt Surg.*, **55B**, 874

Stevens, P. S. (1977). Distal humeral prosthesis for the elbow. *Conference on Joint Replacement of the Upper Limb* (abstracts), Mechanical Engineering Publications Ltd, p. 14

Torgerson, W. R. and Leach, R. E. (1970). Synovectomy of the elbow in rheumatoid arthritis. *J. Bone Jt Surg.*, **52A**, 371

Wilson, D. W., Arden, G. P. and Ansell, B. M. (1973). Synovectomy of the elbow in rheumatoid arthritis. *J. Bone Jt Surg.*, **55B**, 106–111

11

THE WRIST

The wrist includes the radiocarpal, inferior radio-ulnar and intercarpal joints as well as the contents of the extensor and flexor compartments at this level. The wrist joint is frequently the keystone in reconstructive surgery of the hand and provides a sound base upon which satisfactory finger function depends. Its influence on more distal structures may be direct by disturbance of the tendons passing distally over it or indirect by inducing compensatory deformities to its own mal-alignment.

Synovitis, as elsewhere, produces pain and limitation of movement, erosions, deformity and instability or stiffness. The radio-ulnar joint is involved early in the disease with consequent pain on rotation and discomfort on moving the ulnar head relative to the radius (figure 11.1). Local injections of steroid, and splintage may be helpful. Early palmar flexion deformities can be helped by manipulation into dorsiflexion and a short period in a plaster splint.

THE CARPAL TUNNEL

The median nerve

Synovitis of the flexor tendons within the carpal tunnel may produce median nerve compression with consequent paraesthesiae of median nerve distribution which may progress to hypoaesthesia. Later, loss of sensation, wasting and weakness of the thenar muscles occur. Early wasting can be detected by examination of the radial border of the thenar eminence in skyline view and is due to loss of bulk of the abductor pollicis brevis. In rheumatoid arthritis an alternative cause for loss of median nerve function is a perivasculitis of the vessels within the nerve, which accounts for some cases not relieved by surgical decompression of the nerve. Unlike those patients with intraneural fibrosis due to prolonged nerve compression, fascicular dissection is not effective.

The long flexor tendons

These may rupture within the carpal tunnel following synovial compression. Repair is best carried out by synovial clearance and re-attachment of the distal stumps to a suitable intact motor tendon. The most frequently encountered rupture is that of the flexor pollicis longus. This tendon lies on the floor of the carpal tunnel and tends to rupture where it crosses the trapezioscaphoid joint by attrition produced by bony roughness of the

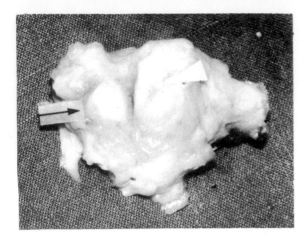

Figure 11.1 There is a considerable synovial fold around the radio-ulnar joint and this is probably why it is involved early

THE EXTENSOR APPARATUS OF THE WRIST

The extensor tendons are ensheathed and lie in separate compartments at the wrist. Individual tendons may rupture as a result of synovial compression and subsequent necrosis (figure 11.2). Inability to extend the fingers may also occur because of dislocation of the extensor tendons ulnarwards off the metacarpal heads, thus producing relative lengthening. A rare cause of dropped fingers is a posterior interosseous nerve palsy. True attrition rupture of the extensors on sharp spikes of bone arising from an eroded head of the ulna also occurs (Vaughan-Jackson, 1948; figure 11.3); the nearest extensor, that of the little finger, is sawn through first and the other extensors are involved in turn (figure 11.4). Prophylactic surgery in the form of decompression of the extensor compartment is valuable (figure 11.5) and may be all that is necessary. However, excision of the synovium, which can be considerable in quantity, is of value in treating the disease in general, for its removal can lead to quiescence of the arthritis. Placement of the extensor retinaculum between the dorsum of the radius and the tendons forms a floor protecting them from the underlying bone, thus diminishing the likelihood of further rupture.

Repair of the ruptured extensor tendons is usually combined with excision of the head of the ulna. To save overloading a solitary motor ten-

joint margin. Rupture of the flexor pollicis longus is one cause of the boutonnière type of Z deformity of the thumb producing flexion at the metacarpophalangeal joint and hyperextension at the interphalangeal joint.

Not infrequently the interphalangeal joint of the thumb is also involved in rheumatoid disease and under those circumstances restoration of function is best achieved by fusion of the interphalangeal joint in 20° flexion. Repair by bridge graft can be effective if the joints are reasonably healthy.

Figure 11.2 This illustrates two mechanisms of tendon rupture in the same patient. (a) Due to impaction of synovium in the extensor retinaculum causing necrosis of the middle two tendons. (b) This was a true attrition rupture due to a rough area of bone on the ulnar head

a

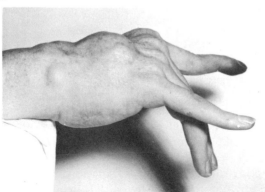

b

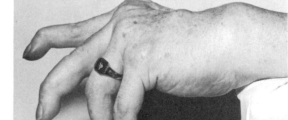

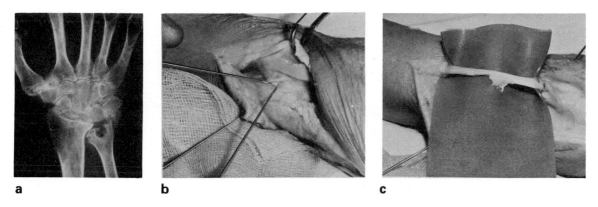

a   b   c

Figure 11.3 (a) The eroded head of the ulna; (b) the dark metal pointer on a sharp spike of bone arising from the head of the ulna; (c) the fraying that has occurred in the tendon about the rupture. (O. Vaughan-Jackson)

don, we frequently employ bridge grafts and despite the double anastomosis these work well (figure 11.6). For rupture of the thumb extensor, transposition of the extensor indicis proprius to serve as its motor is effective. An important operative point is to ensure the repaired extensor holds the metacarpophalangeal joint in 20° more of extension than the normal resting position, otherwise the tendon will be too lax.

DE QUERVAIN'S DISEASE

Stenosis of the fibrous sheath or synovitis of the abductor pollicis longus and the extensor pollicis

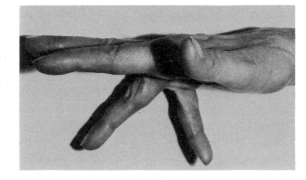

Figure 11.4 Attrition rupture of the little and ring finger extensors

Figure 11.5 (a) Shows the build-up of synovium distal to the extensor retinaculum. (b) It is impaction of this synovium that has caused the ruptures seen here

a   b

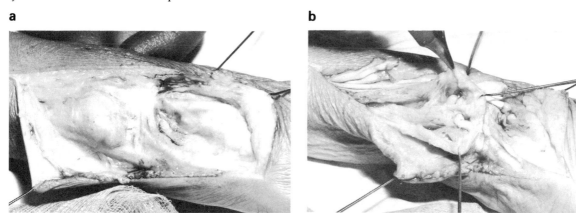

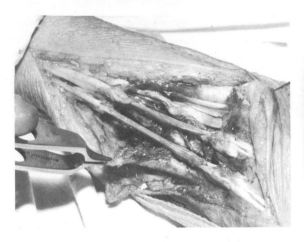

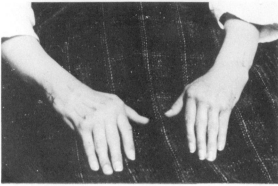

Figure 11.7 The Z deformity

Figure 11.6 Bridge grafting of ruptured tendons

brevis tendons as they pass over the radial styloid may result in pain on thumb movements. Adduction and flexion of the thumb metacarpal exacerbate this pain, and tucking the thumb into the palm while pushing the wrist into ulnar deviation produces the same effect, namely Finkelstein's test. Injections of steroid may result in permanent relief of symptoms. However, recurrence or persistence of symptoms is an indication for surgery. Through a longitudinal incision over the radial styloid, care being taken not to injure the radial nerve, the tendons are decompressed. It must be remembered that the abductor longus tendon may be duplicated and lie in separate compartments. Division of the fibrous sheath and synovectomy effect a cure.

THE Z DEFORMITY

Radial deviation of the wrist, said to occur secondary to rupture of the extensor carpi ulnaris tendon, induces a compensatory ulnar deviation of the fingers at the metacarpophalangeal joints (figure 11.7). Early restoration of the balance of forces by repair of the extensor carpi ulnaris should arrest further progress of the deformity (Vaughan-Jackson and Stack, 1971). In over 100 personal ulnar head excisions, inspection of the ulnar carpal tendons was undertaken routinely and, though often found displaced, they were never found to be ruptured. A helpful manoeuvre to restore balance is transfer of the split extensor

carpi radialis longus tendon to the flexor carpi ulnaris and extensor carpi ulnaris, respectively; this may also prevent volar subluxation. Osteotomy of the radius to correct radial deviation has its advocates (Davidson and Caird, 1976).

Alternatively, if the wrist is badly damaged, arthrodesis of the joint in 15° of ulnar deviation may improve alignment of the fingers.

VOLAR SUBLUXATION OF THE WRIST

This common finding can embarrass long flexor tendons, resulting in pain and loss of function. The deformity can be tackled in two ways. Reduction and temporary fixation by Steinman pins with external splintage for 8 weeks may restore the alignment and also preserve some wrist movement; this procedure has been called fibrous stabilisation of the wrist (Lance, 1975). If cartilage destruction is unlikely to allow an adequate return of function and stability, then wrist fusion or arthroplasty is performed.

ULNAR HEAD EXCISION

Excision of the ulnar head and synovial clearance of the wrist is one of the most rewarding forms of surgery in rheumatoid disease (figure 11.8) (Straub and Ranawat, 1969; Rana and Taylor, 1972; Helal and Mikic, 1973).

In a study of ulnar head excision in 125 wrists of 95 rheumatoid patients (Helal and Mikic) the following conclusions were arrived at:

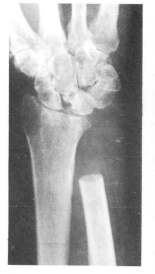 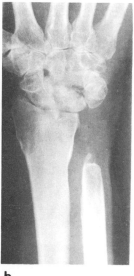

a   **b**

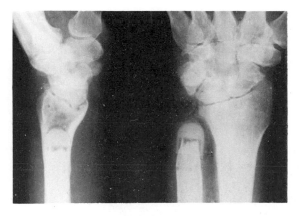

Figure 11.9 In this patient a silastic head was helpful, as too much of the distal end of the ulna had been excised and there was some discomfort over the apex of the stump

Figure 11.8 Eight years have elapsed between photographs (a) and (b). At (a) excision of the head of the ulna was combined with synovectomy of the wrist. Despite progression of the disease elsewhere, including the carpus, excellent function has been maintained in the wrist joint, which remains painless and almost fully mobile

(1) The optimum length of the distal end of the ulna to be excised is between 1 and 1½ cm.

(2) The results were good if the radiocarpal joint was stable, even if it was damaged and stiff.

(3) Removal of the ulnar head did not produce ulnar drift or shift.

(4) Silicone rubber ulnar heads are not necessary and did not seem to improve the outcome (figure 11.9).

(5) Prevention of rupture of extensor tendons, where possible by ulnar head excision or decompression of the extensor compartment, is preferable to repair which does not give perfect results.

(6) The best results from ulnar head excision were those carried out reasonably early and combined with wrist synovectomy.

ARTHRODESIS

Excision of the lower ulna, synovial clearance and rawing of the articular surfaces of the radiocarpal

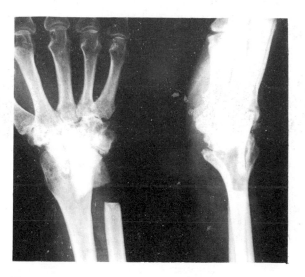

Figure 11.10 Fusion using a tibial graft

int are performed and a gutter cut in the carpus to take a graft running from the middle metacarpal base to the radius. The graft can be taken from the upper tibia (figure 11.10), the lower end of the ulna (figure 11.11) or an iliac bone block (figure 11.12).

At the London Hospital a compression staple devised by W. Day of Imperial College is employed in combination with a Rush nail threaded down one of the metacarpals to stabilise the wrist fusion; excellent fixation is obtained (figure 11.13).

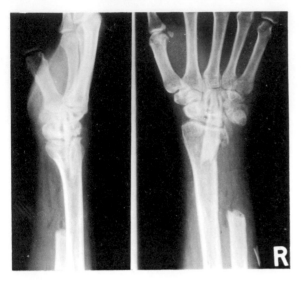

Figure 11.11 In this method of fusion the excised lower end of the ulna is used to provide a graft

Figure 11.12 Fusion using a corticocancellous piece of iliac crest

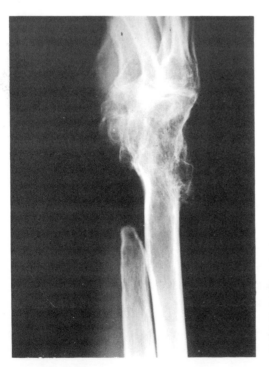

It is generally unnecessary to add bone graft, for if the bones are well coapted, this form of internal fixation is sufficient (figure 1 i.14); however, it is wise to apply external splintage as well. Mannerfelt and Malmsten (1971) have described fixation by a compression staple combined with a Rush nail, and state that external splintage is then unnecessary. The Nissen wedge arthrodesis is also effective (chapter 7). The wrist is usually fused in a neutral position, but if both are to be fused, one should be left in 20° flexion to allow the hand to reach the perineum for toilet purposes.

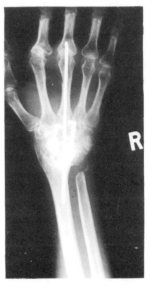
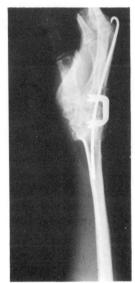

Figure 11.13 London Hospital staple and Rush nail. Mannerfelt type of fusion

Figure 11.14 The compression staple and Rush nail successfully used in the presence of gross loss of bone

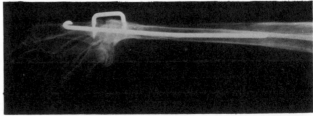

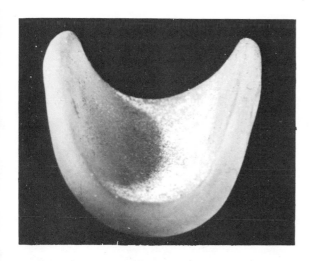

Figure 11.15 Silicone rubber spacer

ARTHROPLASTY OF THE WRIST

If the wrist is stable but stiff because of destruction of the articular surfaces we have employed two procedures. Firstly, an interposition silicone rubber 3 mm spacer, cut from a precurved sheet, is suitable if there is reasonable bony congruity (figure 11.15). Secondly, if the wrist is stable and stiff, with gross distortion of the bony surfaces, the ulnar head is excised and the scaphoid and lunate replaced by rubber prostheses of Swanson design cemented together with silicone rubber adhesive. Of twelve patients who were suitable for a silicone rubber spacer and have more than 2 years' follow-up, seven have regained one-half to three-quarters range of movement; three are stiff but painless; two have some movement with discomfort and have required further surgery.

A Swanson design bi-stemmed wrist prosthesis of silicone rubber is also available; he reports good results following its use (figure 11.16).

Several other new artificial wrist joints have been described, notably by Meuli (1973), and by

Gschwend, Scheier and Bahler (1977), Greenwald *et al.* (1977) and Lennox (1977). Most experience has been with the Meuli design (figure 11.17).

The Meuli wrist arthroplasty (Meuli, 1973) has a ball-and-socket design. The ball is attached on a trunnion located by a stem in the radius, and the socket has two stems which pass into the shafts of the appropriate metacarpals, usually the index and middle. The stems can be offset by bending and can be cemented into place.

A 2-year follow-up of 26 wrist arthroplasties in 22 patients has been reported; re-operation was necessary in 35 per cent of the cases due to neglecting to place the centre of rotation in the capitate area, resulting in a tendency to flexion and ulnar deviation; 77 per cent of the results after re-operation were considered good (Beckenbaugh and Linscheid, 1977).

SURGICAL TECHNIQUE; A FEW SUGGESTIONS

Straight incisions are preferred, as curved incisions may be undermined, with consequent wound breakdown and often skin necrosis. Dorsal approaches are recommended for extensor compartment synovectomy, wrist arthroplasty and wrist fusions. A dorso-ulnar approach over the head of the ulna is recommended for its excision, and a radial approach for decompression of tendons over the radial styloid. It must be remembered that the extensor pollicis longus tendon crosses obliquely to its tunnel, and, unless identified and followed, can easily be cut accidentally, as it lies buried in a mass of synovitis. When inserting a Rush nail for wrist arthrodesis, it is introduced into the most appropriate metacarpal in line with the radial shaft. When replacing the proximal row of the carpus with a silastic scapho-lunate prosthesis, it is important to close the capsule thoroughly for stability.

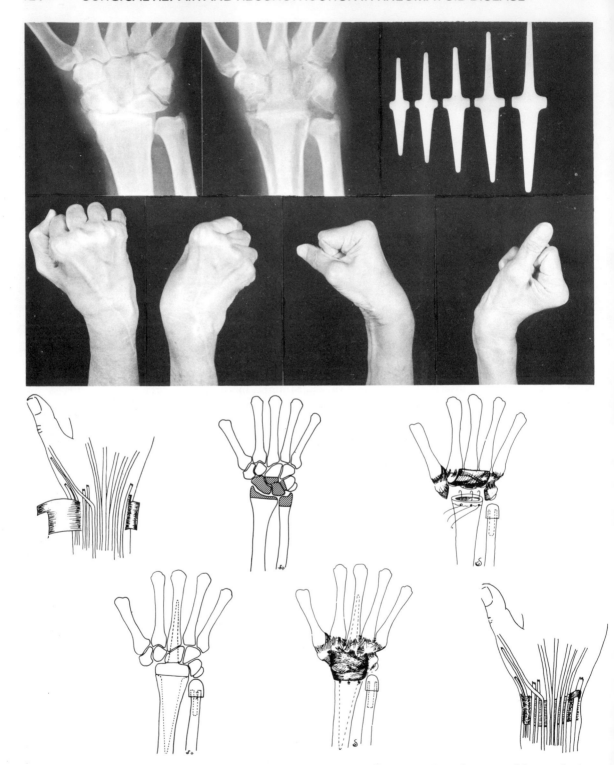

Figure 11.16 Swanson bistemmed silicone prosthesis showing required bone resection, placement of the prosthesis, X-rays and the clinical pictures of the range of movement (A. Swanson)

Figure 11.17 Meuli design of total wrist replacement

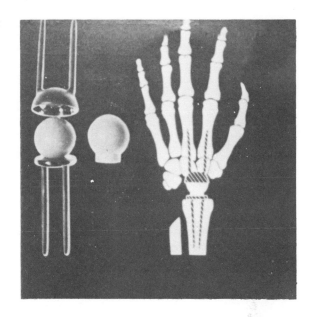

REFERENCES

Beckenbaugh, R. D. and Linscheid, R. L. (1977). Total wrist arthroplasty. *J. Hand Surg.*, **2**, No. 5, 337–344

Davidson, E. P. and Caird, D. M. (1976). Osteotomy of the radius in rheumatoid disease, Paper read at *Br. Orth. Ass. Meeting*

Finkelstein, H. (1930). Stenosing tenovaginitis at the radial styloid process. *J. Bone Jt Surg.*, **12**, 509

Greenwald, A. S., Matejczyk, M-B, Porrit, D. S., Wilde, A. H. and Culver, J. E. (1977). Design, development and clinical application of a total wrist replacement. *Conference on Joint Replacement in the Upper Limb* (abstracts), Mechanical Engineering Publications, London

Gschwend, N., Scheier, H. and Bähler, A. (1977). GSB elbow, wrist, MP and PIP joints, *Conference on Joint Replacement in the Upper Limb* (abstracts), Mechanical Engineering Publications, London

Helal, B. and Mikic, Z. (1973). Survey of ulnar head excision and synovectomy, Paper read at *Rheum. Arth. Surg. Soc.*

Lance, E. M. (1975). Fibrous stabilization of the rheumatoid wrist – an alternative to arthrodesis. *S. Afr. Med. J.*, **49**, 1712

Lennox, W. M. (1977). A new prosthesis for the rheumatoid wrist. *Conference on Joint Replacement in the Upper Limb* (abstracts), Mechanical Engineering Publications, London

Mannerfelt, L. and Malmsten, M. (1971). Arthrodesis of the wrist in rheumatoid arthritis, a technique without external fixation. *Scand. J. Plastic Reconstruct. Surg.*, **5**, 124–130

Meuli, H. C. (1973). Arthroplastie du poignet. *Ann. Chir.*, **27**, 527–530

Rana, N. A. and Taylor, A. R. (1972). Excision of the distal end of the ulna in rheumatoid arthritis. *J. Bone Jt Surg.*, **54B**, 169–170

Straub, L. R. and Ranawat, C. S. (1969). The wrist in rheumatoid arthritis. *J. Bone Jt Surg.*, **51A**, 1–20

Swanson, A. (1973). *Flexible Implant Arthroplasty in the Hand and Extremities*, Mosby St. Louis

Vaughan-Jackson, O. J. (1948). Rupture of extensor tendons by attrition at the inferior radioulnar joint. *J. Bone Jt Surg.*, **30B**, 528

Vaughan-Jackson, O. J. and Stack, G. (1971). The zig-zag deformity in the rheumatoid hand. *Hand*, March, 62

12
THE HAND

Patients with rheumatoid disease will tolerate gross dysfunction because the disease progresses at a rate which allows them to accommodate to their disability and, apart from episodes of acute synovitis, pain is not a prominent feature. Patients nevertheless will often attend early for a disfiguring lump such as a rheumatoid nodule on the skin (figure 12.1).

PATTERNS OF DISEASE

There are four different patterns of disease in the hand.

(1) The disease may involve primarily the synovium of the flexor apparatus with virtually no damage or destruction to other structures (figure 12.2).

(2) The synovitis may involve merely the dorsal extensor compartment and joints (figure 12.3).

(3) In the 'fibrotic' type of hand, contracted soft tissues produce deformity and loss of movement (figure 12.4).

(4) In the neuropathic type of hand, the joints undergo bone absorption resulting in unrestricted mobility and joint instability is the main feature (figure 12.5).

An infinite variety of patterns of disease are produced by mixtures of these pathologies.

ASSESSMENT AND PRIORITIES IN RHEUMATOID HAND SURGERY

It cannot be too strongly emphasised that surgery should only be carried out to prevent impending dysfunction or to improve function and to this end a thorough and meticulous assessment has to be made. A similar assessment after operation will prove an accurate guide to the results achieved. A detailed and quantitative assessment requires more time than a clinician can spare in a busy outpatients clinic and thus examination is carried out and recorded by occupational therapists, who can also observe the patients in their home environment. The evidence they collect guides the surgeon comprehensively in assessing the patient's problems. Sometimes a simple mechanical aid will achieve the desired functional improvement and surgery can then be delayed indefinitely.

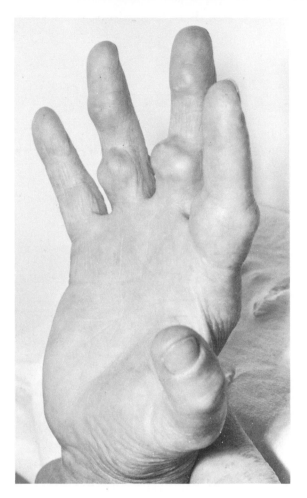

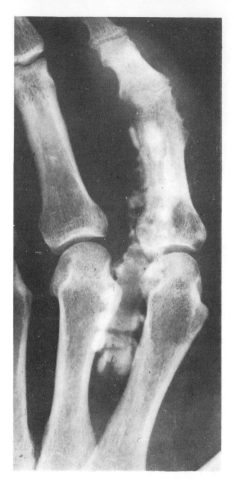

Figure 12.1 Rheumatoid nodules on the skin. Patients may attend early because of disfigurement

Figure 12.2 Tenograph of synovitis of the flexor apparatus. There is no other problem in this rheumatoid hand

Careful consideration must be given to priorities in carrying out surgery for multiple hand deformities. The first priority is decompression and synovectomy of tendon sheaths to prevent rupture of tendons. Of second priority is synovectomy of joints in which the deformity is incipient. The lowest degree of priority is given to established deformities.

In dealing with established deformities it is a good rule to operate on one hand at a time, and if thumb and fingers require surgery, to deal with the thumb first and separately from other portions of the hand. By so doing, the patient can keep the hand in use and regain early independence following surgery.

SOFT TISSUE SWELLINGS

Soft tissue swellings are of two types: either rheumatoid nodules located immediately beneath the skin, or synovial swellings that arise from the synovial linings of joints, tendons and bursae.

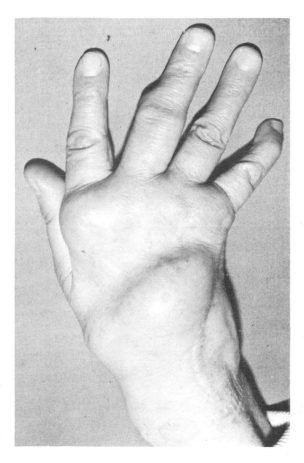

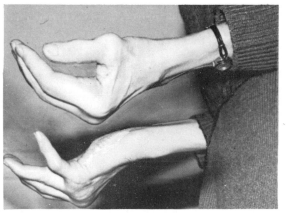

Figure 12.4 The fibrotic rheumatoid hand. Loss of movement is the key feature

Figure 12.3 Synovial swellings. These are arising from the inferior radio-ulnar joint, the extensor tendons, the metacarpophalangeal joints and the proximal interphalangeal joint of the middle finger

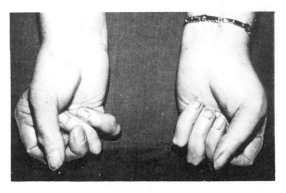

Figure 12.5 The neuropathic hand. Movement is good. Painless instability is the key feature

Rheumatoid nodules

Nodules which are tender and cause necrosis of the overlying skin should be excised. Excision must be complete, and when associated with underlying bursae, the latter should also be excised totally. Utmost gentleness and thorough haemostasis are essential, especially when the patient is on steroids, to avoid the troublesome triad of haematoma, wound breakdown and infection.

Synovial swellings

It may be necessary to excise the synovium of the underlying joint or tendons to cure these.

SYNOVITIS

The flexor apparatus

The flexor tendons may be embarrassed by synovitis, at various levels and in varying degrees of severity. The most common lesion is triggering at metacarpal head level; less frequently appreciated is the similar problem at proximal interphalangeal joint level (Helal, 1969; 1970; 1974). When severe this results in gross loss of flexion; even passive flexion of the proximal interphalangeal joint is

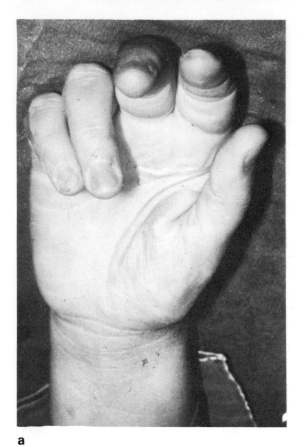
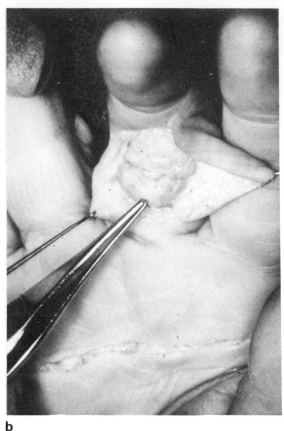

a   b

Figure 12.6   Entrapment of the profundus in the index and middle finger results in gross loss of flexion; (b) marked synovitis of the flexors in the region of the proximal interphalangeal joint

blocked. Three mechanisms of proximal interphalangeal joint obstruction are recognised:

(1) Synovitis with ballooning through the thinner wall of the sheath overlying the joint (figure 12.6).

(2) Adhesions between the sublimis and the profundus.

(3) A nodule on the profundus tendon preventing normal passage through the sublimis decussation (figure 12.7). The diagnostic sign is loss of active flexion at the terminal joint when the proximal joint is passively fully flexed (usually a maximum of 90° or less) (figure 12.8). Treatment consists of surgical synovial clearance of the flexor sheath, leaving a bridge over the proximal phalanx. Occasionally the ulnar slip of the sublimis may have to be excised to allow easy passage of the

profundus through the decussation. Nodules on the flexor tendon are generally due to synovial intrusion at the level of the vinculae where there is a normal invagination of the visceral layer of synovium.

Rupture of the long flexors in the hand generally occurs at the proximal limit of the fibrous flexor sheath or within the carpal tunnel, and is associated with compression of the tendon by synovium (figure 12.9). Repair of flexor tendon ruptures carries a worse prognosis than in the non-rheumatoid patient because of the friable state of the tendons, which do not hold sutures well. Also, the necessary immobilisation to allow healing results in deleterious stiffening of finger joints.

Sublimis transfer from the middle to the ring finger or from the ring to the little finger is one of the most successful manoeuvres; care must be taken to stabilise the volar aspect of the proximal joint of the donor digit by tenodesis of one of the sublimis slips in order to prevent a swan-neck deformity occurring. For tendon grafting, our experience has shown that fascia lata strips appear to be the most valuable donor material. The results of two-stage silastic grafting and of using artificial tendons are not satisfactory, and not infrequently the best solution, especially when joint damage coexists, is to perform arthrodesis of the interphalangeal joints in the optimum position.

Synovitis of the joints

This may result in pain, swelling, stiffness, joint destruction and instability. If the synovitis does not resolve within 12 weeks of medical treatment or if it is causing persistent pain, synovectomy should be performed. Ideally, synovectomy should be undertaken before loss of joint space, erosions or instability appear. There is little doubt that pain is relieved and joint function temporarily restored. It is important for the long-term assessment of results that immediate post-operative X-

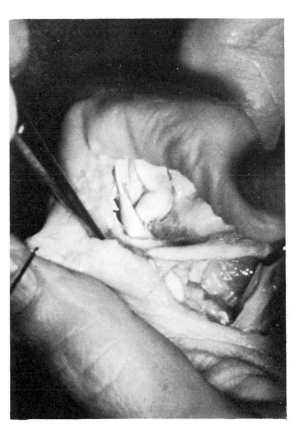

Figure 12.8 The sign of 'distal' entrapment of the flexor tendons. On flexing the proximal joint passively to the maximum, here limited to 90°, active flexion of the terminal joint is abolished

Figure 12.7 A nodule on the profundus blocking excursion of the tendon through the sublimis decussation

Figure 12.9 Rupture of the flexors of the little finger at the point of their entry into the flexor sheath

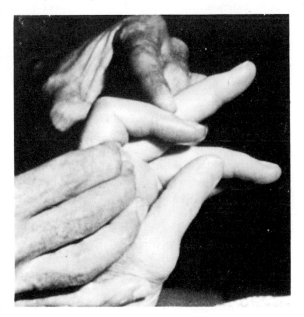

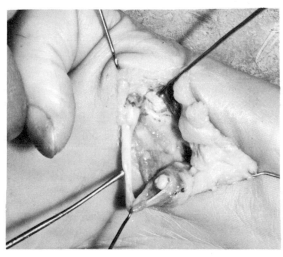

rays are taken. The clearance of synovium which has eroded bone recently may take with it bone debris, which in pre-operative X-rays is sufficiently radio-opaque to mask erosions (figure 12.10). The progress of local joint disease may be arrested by synovectomy; evidence is conflicting. An alternative method of treatment has been described by Benjamin (1976) for the metacarpophalangeal joints, and consists of an osteotomy proximal and distal to the joint. After 10 years experience the results are very satisfactory (figure 12.11; chapter 5).

THE JOINTS

The functionally significant joints of the hand are the carpometacarpal of the thumb joint and all the metacarpophalangeal and interphalangeal joints. These joints and the muscles acting upon them, are an interlinked mechanism; the normal posture and activity is the outcome of finely balanced forces acting upon this system. Disorder of muscle action, of capsule, of ligaments, of synovium, of cartilage and of bone all contribute to the varying pattern of pathology and deformity typical of rheumatoid disease in the hand.

Subluxation or dislocation of joints occurs because those structures that normally resist displacement are damaged, namely articular cartilage, subchondral bone, capsule and ligaments. However, the deformity depends on the balance of forces acting upon the joint; these are external, such as the push of opposing digits or gravity, and internal, namely the pull of muscles. Muscle imbalance may arise in the following ways:

(1) Tendons may be directly embarrassed by synovitis, displaced by joint swelling or subluxation, or ruptured by the sharp bony margins of an eroded joint or by synovial impaction.

(2) The motor nerve to the muscle may be compressed by synovial swelling. Common sites for nerve compression are the ulnar nerve in its tunnel at the elbow, the posterior interosseus nerve in the supinator and the ulnar and median nerves in their tunnels at the wrist. Nerve conduction may be disturbed by ischaemia due to arteritis of the vasa nervorum.

(3) Rarely, muscle fibre can be involved when its blood supply is affected by rheumatoid arteritis. However, in practice it is unusual to find any abnormality of the muscle itself apart from disuse atrophy.

FINGER DEFORMITIES IN RHEUMATOID ARTHRITIS

Ulnar drift

Many theories as to the causation of ulnar drift have been mooted:

(1) The anatomical arrangement of ligaments allows the metacarpophalangeal joints to deviate ulnarwards more than radially.

(2) In the 'armchair' position gravity pulls the fingers ulnarwards.

(3) In power grip the fingers are forced ulnarwards by the thumb.

(4) The general pull of the long tendons is ulnarwards.

(5) There is a thinner dorsal capsule on the radial than on the ulnar side of the joint, so that synovial protrusion will tend to balloon proximal to the extensor hood on the radial side. As the finger extends, the extensor hood moves proximally; this movement is blocked on the radial side but continues on the ulnar side, thus pulling the proximal phalanx ulnarwards (figure 12.12).

(6) Radial deviation of the wrist may cause secondary ulnar deviation of the fingers (figure 12.13).

Once ulnar deviation has occurred, all the forces acting across the joint tend to increase the deformity. Splintage is mandatory after any surgical correction but is of little value therapeutically, although it may help to prevent the ulnar drift from worsening while the patient awaits surgery. It is difficult to sort out primary causes from secondary effects. For example, there is almost invariably ulnar dislocation of the extensor and flexor tendons, and some degree of volar subluxation of the proximal phalanx in relation to the metacarpal head. Thus two factors seem indispensable to ulnar drift: firstly, instability of the

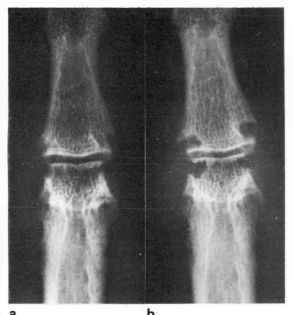

a   **b**

Figure 12.10 (a) Before and (b) after synovectomy. Erosions not visible pre-operatively have become apparent on an immediate post-operative X-ray as synovial cavities containing bone debris have been surgically cleared

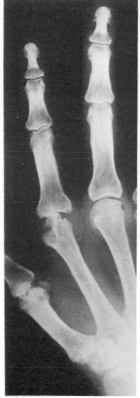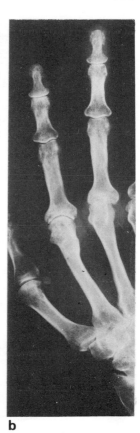

a   **b**

Figure 12.11 Before and after Benjamin osteotomy. Metacarpophalangeal double osteotomy, index finger only: (a) immediately before operation in 1968; (b) 7 years later

metacarpophalangeal joints, and secondly, intact long tendons. It is interesting to note that ulnar drift does not occur in digits in which the flexors and extensors have been divided—for example, in traumatic amputation of the terminal phalanx; nor does it occur if rupture of the flexor apparatus precedes the deformity in the other digits. Early radial deviation of the wrist can be corrected by transfer of the extensor carpi radialis longus to the ulnar side of the wrist. Correction of the ulnar drift, in the early stages, may be accomplished by synovial clearance of the metacarpophalangeal joints and relocation of the extensor tendons by releasing the dorsal capsule on the ulnar side and by reefing it on the radial side. This repair can be further reinforced by rerouting the extensor indicis proprius tendon to the radial side of the proximal phalanx (figure 12.14). In established cases of marked ulnar drift with good preservation of the metacarpophalangeal joints the following procedure is valuable.

The indicis proprius tendon is looped around the lumbrical tendon and brought back to be sutured to the extensor apparatus as far distally as possible. In the ulnar three digits the radial half of the respective extensor digitorum tendon is detached at mid-proximal phalangeal level and dissected back to mid-metacarpal level, looped around the transverse metacarpal ligament and resutured to its parent extensor as far distally as possible (figure 12.15). Several other forms of repair, generally by transposing the intrinsic muscles, are described but do not usually work as well. If there is considerable articular damage or volar subluxation, or both, then reconstruction is best answered by arthroplasty of the metacarpophalangeal joint. Ulnar drift can be corrected

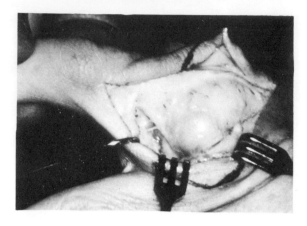

Figure 12.12 Synovium protrusion on the radial side has blocked proximal movement of the extensor expansion. Unrestricted movement on the ulnar side causes ulnar deviation

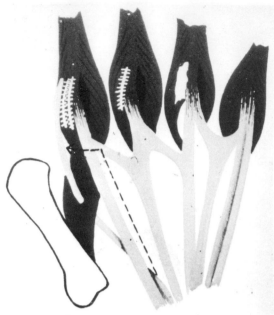

Figure 12.14 Ulnar drift correction by ulnar side release and radial reefing of the dorsal capsule and the extensor indicis proprius is moved to the radial side of the joint

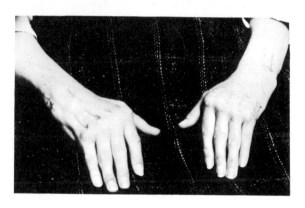

Figure 12.13 Ulnar drift secondary to radial deviation of the wrist which in turn occurred because of displacement of the ulnar carpal tendons

also by osteotomy and this method is under trial (figure 12.16).

Excision arthroplasty, while often producing satisfactory results, can be enhanced by using joint spacers. Two 'integral hinge' joint replacements are in common use: the Swanson (1972) joint and the Calnan–Nicolle joint (Nicolle and Calnan, 1972). Good results can be achieved using either, the advantages of the latter include built-in collateral stability and a capsular bulb, which prevents encroachment of fibrous tissue, producing a smooth and more natural outline to the joint.

Although the polypropylene hinge tends to fracture, this may produce no particular problem, since the fibrous capsule around the prosthesis maintains the joint space. Other prosthetic joints are still at the 'experimental' stage.

The Boutonnière deformity

This combines flexion deformity at the proximal and hyperextension at the distal interphalangeal joint (figure 12.17). The cause is synovitis of the proximal joint, which either stretches or ruptures the extensor tendon middle slip insertion into the base of the middle phalanx, and which is normally responsible for extending this phalanx. In the early stages synovectomy of the proximal joint and splintage will correct the deformity; unfortunately, the repair suitable in a purely traumatic boutonnière with an otherwise normal hand, (figure 12.18) is sometimes unsuccessful in rheumatoid cases. Elongation of the extensor tendon over the middle phalanx will

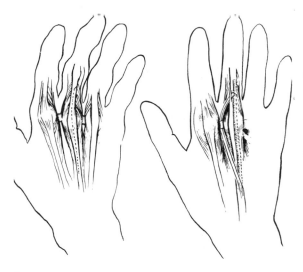

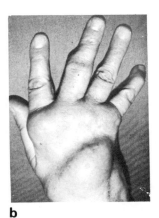

a

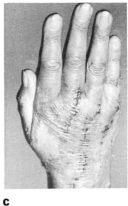

b   **c**

Figure 12.15 (a) Technique for correction of ulnar drift. (b) Pre-operative appearances. (c) After syno-vectomy of metacarpophalangeal joints and extensor 'loop' procedure

correct the accompanying hyperextension of the terminal joint and will improve the functional position of the finger. Of the reconstructive techniques the best is that of Matev (1964) (figure 12.18). It is essential to overcome any fixed flexion deformity by an Odstock spring splint (figure 3.15a, p. 36). Replacement of the proximal joint by a spacer, or by fusion of the joint using a Harrison–Nicolle (1972) peg are the final salvage procedures.

The swan-neck deformity

This combines hyperextension at the proximal and a flexion deformity at the distal interphalangeal joint. The flexion deformity of the terminal joint is due to a relative increase in pull of the flexor brought about by the extended proximal interphalangeal joint and frequently by concurrent volar subluxation of the metacarpophalangeal joint (figure 12.19). In this deformity the forces acting on the proximal interphalangeal joint have an extensor preponderance and the causes in order of frequency are:

(1) Tightness of the intrinsic muscle tendon often brought about by synovitis or by the volar displacement of the metacarpophalangeal joint. To test for intrinsic tightness, the range of passive flexion in the proximal joint is measured with the metacarpophalangeal joint in extension and then in flexion, thus separating the origin and insertion of the muscle and bringing the origin and insertion close together. The first position will reduce the range; the second will allow more flexion at the proximal joint. In the absence of secondary contractures of the capsule and ligaments of the proximal joint, the following procedures will improve the deformity: Littler's release, which is division of the intrinsic muscle tendons (figure 12.20), and Zancolli's release, which mobilises the two extensor slips and allows them to drop volarwards on either side of the joint. This last procedure is the one of choice in the early stages of deformity.

(2) Rupture or displacement of the flexor sub-limis tendon reduces flexor action on the proximal joint, thus shifting the balance of forces in favour of the extensor. Synovectomy or repair of the ruptured tendon will correct this.

(3) Overaction of the extensor middle slip sometimes occurs after too tight an extensor repair (figure 12.21) or rupture of the extensor attachment to the terminal phalanx, allowing the full force of extensor action to fall on the middle phalanx. Readjustment of the extensor apparatus will correct these faults. This type of swan-neck deformity gives rise to a paradoxical sign contrasting with intrinsic tightness, for extension of the metacarpophalangeal joints will, by relaxing the

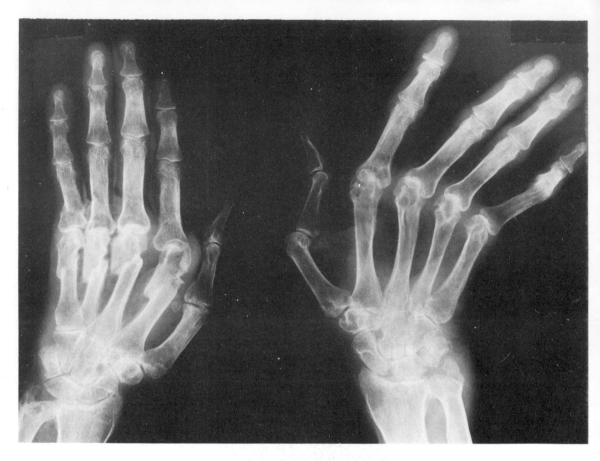

Figure 12.16 Ulnar drift correction by osteotomy

extensor, allow more flexion at the proximal interphalangeal joint.

(4) The volar plate of the proximal joint may rupture or be stretched by synovitis of the proximal joint, or be involved secondarily to one of the above causes of swan-neck deformity. The plate normally acts as a check to hyperextension of the proximal joint. To correct this form of swan-neck deformity, the contracted portions of the capsule are excised and the volar plate is reinforced by a tenodesis using one of the slips of sublimis (Littler, 1964).

Secondary contracture of the collateral ligaments and lateral capsule can occur and will perpetuate the deformity. Progressive surgical release of the capsular structures is carried out, starting on the dorsal surface and working palmarwards until adequate flexion is achieved. Silas-

tic membranes can be interposed between dorsal tendons and joint to prevent re-adhesion.

The Mallet deformity

Spontaneous rupture of the extensor at its insertion into the terminal phalanx occurs rarely in

Figure 12.17 Boutonnière deformity due to rupture of the middle slip of the extensor to the middle finger

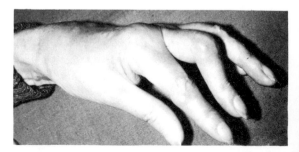

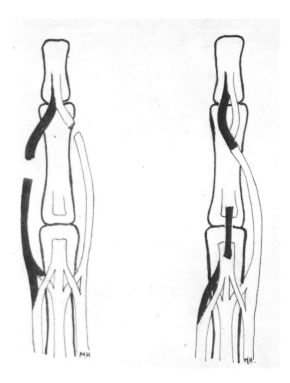

Figure 12.18 Matev repair for boutonnière

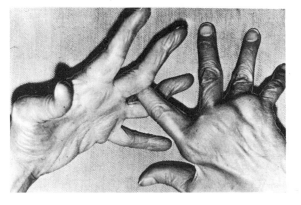

Figure 12.19 Swan neck deformity. In this instance there is volar subluxation of the metacarpophalangeal joint which stretches the intrinsics, producing a 'tightness'

rheumatoid disease; if it does, the tendon usually reattaches itself satisfactorily with or without a suitable support such as an Oakley splint (figure 12.22). If this treatment fails the method described by Iselin is sometimes effective: an ellipse of skin and tendon on the dorsum of the terminal joint is excised, followed by suture of tendon and skin together in one layer.

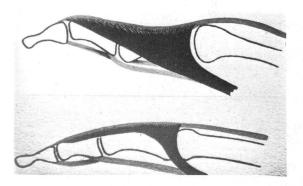

Figure 12.20 Littler's release of intrinsic tightness

JOINT REPLACEMENT IN THE HAND

Factors extrinsic to the joint are often responsible for limitation of joint movement and deformity, particularly at the proximal interphalangeal joint. This is demonstrated by the fact that adequate removal of bone by arthroplasty or a telescoping osteotomy, of the metacarpal will, by relaxation of soft tissues, often result in functional improvement of the other joints in the same digit. Accurate diagnosis is paramount to successful management.

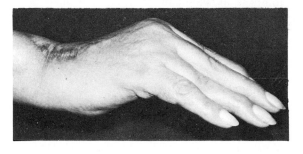

Figure 12.21 Swan neck deformity due to extensor adhesions

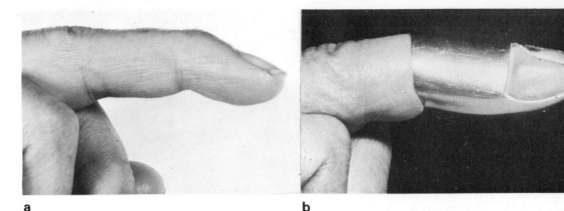

a   b

Figure 12.22 (a) Mallet deformity. (b) Mallet deformity treated by Oakley splint

Limited destructive changes can be an indication for refashioning of the joint surface and perichondrial grafting; perichondrium is stripped from the rib cartilage and the deep surface faced towards the joint cavity.

Arthroplasty of the metacarpophalangeal joints

Replacement is usually carried out for gross instability or stiffness.

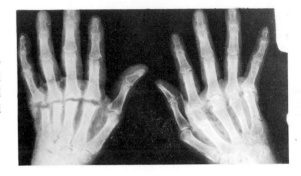

Figure 12.23 Simple excision arthroplasty of metacarpophalangeal joints

Excision arthroplasty

Excision arthroplasty of the metacarpophalangeal joints is indicated in patients with small bones whose medullae are too narrow to accept a stemmed prosthesis, and moderately good function can be achieved (figure 12.23).

Replacement arthroplasty

A variety of prostheses are available for the replacement of metacarpophalangeal and proximal interphalangeal joints (figure 12.24) but a perfect prosthesis for these joints has yet to be devised. Many require cement, which adds to the risk of wound breakdown and infection associated with its use in a superficial site; salvage, if necessary, is very difficult. Dacron-covered prostheses which bind into the medullae of the bones

can also cause problems when revision is necessary, due to the difficulty of their removal. Soft spacers (Swanson) provide little collateral stability and there is a tendency for the space created to diminish as fibrous tissue contracts, leading to loss of movement (figure 12.25). Alternatively, if the joints remain mobile, there is a tendency for ulnar drift to recur, which is the bugbear of metacarpophalangeal joint arthroplasty. Reliance should never be placed on the prosthesis alone and soft tissue correction of ulnar drift should always accompany the arthroplasty. Problems with all-metal hinge prostheses in rheumatoid disease arise because lateral and rotating forces are imparted to the stems, which are embedded in poor-quality porotic bone, causing them to loosen and cut out. The Swanson prosthesis acts simply as a spacer, and although some good results are obtained, recurrence of stiffness or instability may occur. The Calnan–Nicolle type has a bulb of silicone rubber

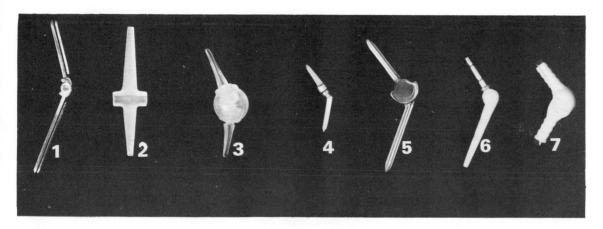

Figure 12.24 Various finger joints: (1) Flatt; (2) Swanson; (3) Calnan–Nicolle; (4) Helal; (5) Devas; (6) St George; (7) Mathys

membrane which prevents fibrosis encroaching on the integral polypropylene hinge and has given reasonable results at the metacarpophalangeal joint (figure 12.26). A degree of collateral stability is provided by the integral hinge and the bulb acts as a soft spacer compressing and expanding with flexion extension movements of the fingers. The bulbs give a more natural outline reproducing the knuckle feature of the hand and are a saving grace of the prosthesis, since the polypropylene frequently breaks. However, provided the prosthesis has been in place for 3 months, a pseudocapsule forms round the silicone rubber bulb and imparts stability with good joint function even if the prosthesis breaks. The non-constrained ICLH (Imperial College London Hospital) prosthesis (figure 12.27) provides a satisfactory spacer but does not prevent a recurrence of ulnar drift. Attempts to build in a Dacron ligament spanning the joint from bone to bone met with little success, since the material is much stronger than the adjacent bone and eventually cuts through it. It is probable that silicone rubber will ultimately prove to be the best material for joint replacements in the hand.

Arthroplasty of the interphalangeal joints

Localising the cause of dysfunction at these joints is difficult. Loss of movement due to tightness

Figure 12.25 Swanson metacarpophalangeal arthroplasty

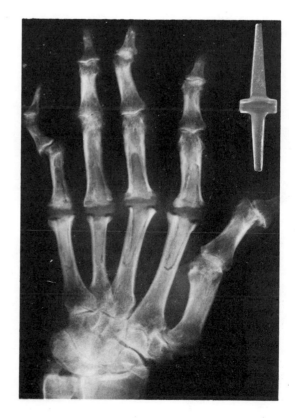

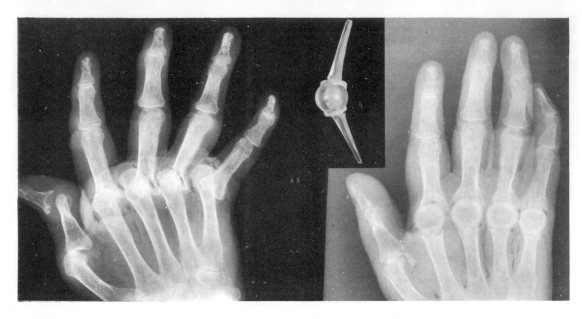

Figure 12.26 Calnan–Nicolle metacarpophalangeal joints

Figure 12.27 ICLH prosthesis (a) before and (b) after operation

a

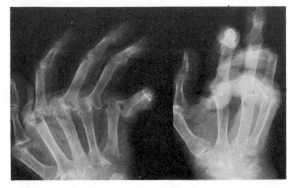

b

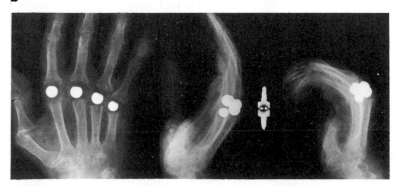

of the various extensor elements acting on the joints has been described and the physical signs outlined. It is, however, often difficult to discover whether capsular contracture or adhesions within the joint cavity are limiting movement. Gross destruction of the articular surface is not infrequently accompanied by a full range of normal movement in addition to adventitious movement, and under these circumstances reasonable function is often retained. Since there is no way of clinically differentiating between the capsular and intra-articular causes of stiffness, it has been our practice to carry out a capsular release as described in swan-neck deformity (Curtis, 1969)

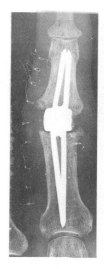
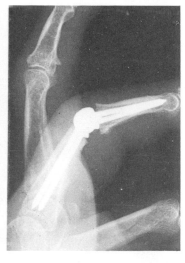

Figure 12.28 Flatt prosthesis provides good stability but the anchorage is apt to cut out of porotic bone

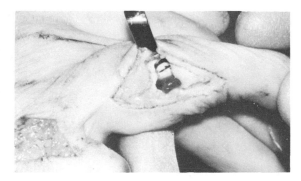

Figure 12.29 The proximal interphalangeal joint prosthesis is introduced through an ulnar side mid-lateral approach

before proceeding. The approach for arthroplasty is from the ulnar side.

Choice of arthroplasty

Many joints are in current use. The metal hinge joint designed by Flatt (1963) (figure 12.28) can be faulted for the same reasons as those of the metacarpophalangeal joint. The Calnan—Nicolle prosthesis is faulted in this situation because of its bulk, which keeps the soft tissue more firmly stretched than one would like in such a restricted situation. The best choice for this joint is the Swanson prosthesis, which acts simply as a spacer. This prosthesis is introduced through an ulnar midlateral approach, which avoids endangering the central middle slip of the extensor, sometimes tenuously attached in rheumatoid disease (Helal, 1967, 1969; figure 12.29). Excellent results can be obtained provided careful selection of patient and joint is made. Post-operatively, splintage and supervised exercises are recommended.

ARTHRODESIS

In the presence of multiple flexor tendon ruptures and damage to the proximal joints, arthrodesis of the latter is the treatment of choice. Harrison and

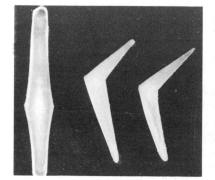
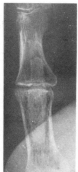

Figure 12.30 Harrison—Nicolle prosthesis for arthrodesis. In this case the metcarpophalangeal thumb joint has not fused by bone

Nicolle (1974) have devised a small peg prosthesis to facilitate this arthrodesis (figure 12.30). The prostheses, made of polypropylene, range from straight (180°) to angles of 20°, 30°, 40° and 50°, thus the desired angle of fusion can be preselected. Although fusion is initially fibrous, it is painless and within months may convert to a bony arthrodesis.

THE RHEUMATOID THUMB

The carpometacarpal is the most important of the thumb joints since it participates in virtually all hand movements. Disease of this joint gives rise to

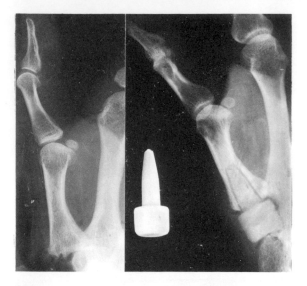

Figure 12.31 Replacement of trapezium by Swanson prosthesis provides arthroplasty of the first carpometacarpal

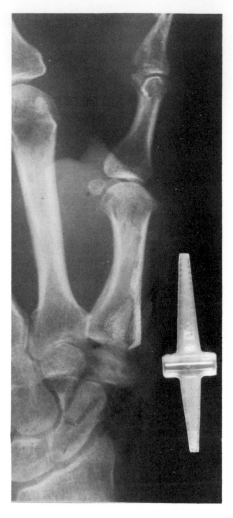

Figure 12.32 A bistemmed Swanson finger joint used as a replacement for the first carpometacarpal joint

pain, stiffness or subluxation. Arthrodesis is unwise, for a pseudoarthrosis formed by excision of the metacarpal base or the trapezium will relieve symptoms and restore function. The results can be embellished by implanting a silicone rubber spacer to maintain thumb length. The Swanson trapezium prosthesis does not seat itself very satisfactorily in a number of cases, and tends to displace, even when reinforced by a loop of abductor tendon (figure 12.31). The Caffiniere prosthesis is a metal on polythene prosthesis, which requires to be implanted into the often porotic rheumatoid bone, and is therefore more troublesome to salvage and should not be employed in the rheumatoid. Interposition arthroplasties, using thin discs of silicone rubber (Kessler, 1973) in the carpometacarpal joint, have not produced good mobility, as they do not create sufficient clearance and the scaphotrapezial joint is often involved. We have been most satisfied with replacement of the trapezium by a Swanson-type finger joint, although the advantage of replacement over simple excision is marginal. One stem is placed in the first metacarpal shaft and the other into a cavity drilled into the scaphoid (figure 12.32). Sometimes adductor release is necessary to mobilise a long-standing adduction deformity.

The metacarpophalangeal joint, if unstable, is best treated by fusion. The surfaces are rawed and apposition is maintained by insertion of a Harrison–Nicolle peg. External splintage for 6 weeks is recommended if the bones are porotic and thin.

Interphalangeal joint instability and deformity are best managed by fusion with a Harrison–Nicolle peg. Kirschner wires, if used, should be parallel, as, if crossed, they will sometimes hold the surfaces apart (figure 12.33).

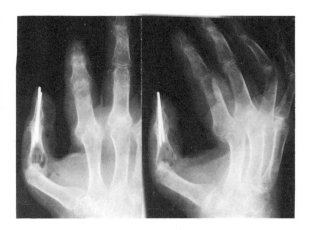

Figure 12.33 Kirschner wires should be put in parallel when used to hold the position for arthrodesis

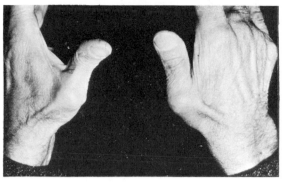

Figure 12.34 Boutonnière of thumb; the displacement of the extensors is well shown

The 'hitch-hiker' or 'Z' deformity of the thumb

This comprises a flexion deformity of the metacarpophalangeal joint and a hyperextension of the interphalangeal joint of the thumb. There are two ways in which this can be produced:

(1) Most frequently, it is associated with boutonnière deformity. Synovitis of the metacarpophalangeal joint displaces the long and short extensors, the long extensor being displaced ulnarwards into the first web space and the short, radialwards, the metacarpal prolapses dorsally between them (figure 12.34). The now unresisted pull of the flexor brevis, the adductor and the short abductor flexes the proximal phalanx and a compensatory hyperextension of the interphalangeal joint occurs. A repair can be effected by transposing the abductor pollicis longus and extensor pollicis brevis tendons just proximal to the metacarpophalangeal joint; the abductor is used as the motor for the distal part of the extensor and the extensor as the motor for the abductor; at the same time it is possible to lengthen the long extensor. If the interphalangeal joint is subluxed and unstable, it should be arthrodesed and the extensor mechanism transferred to an insertion on the proximal phalanx.

(2) More rarely, the deformity arises because the flexor pollicis longus ruptures in the carpal tunnel as it passes over a sharp bony edge on the scaphotrapezial joint; a true attrition rupture. Direct repair is satisfactory if the interphalangeal joint is healthy; otherwise arthrodesis of the interphalangeal joint with the joint in 20° flexion will rebalance the thumb.

The swan-neck thumb

This is a hyperextension deformity of the metacarpophalangeal joint and a flexion deformity of the interphalangeal joint. The deformity is invariably associated with arthritis of the carpometacarpal joint, with adduction and flexion of the first metacarpal. The hyperextension of the metacarpophalangeal and the flexion of the interphalangeal joints are compensatory to accommodate thumb function (figure 12.35). Arthroplasty of the carpometacarpal joint and, if necessary, soft tissue release to allow abduction and extension of the first metacarpal, with stabilisation of the metacarpophalangeal joint by a Harrison–Nicolle peg, restores excellent function.

OPERATIVE TECHNIQUES

Approaches:

(1) To the flexor apparatus. The best exposure is provided by the Bruner 'Z' incision, which passes diagonally across the digit between one

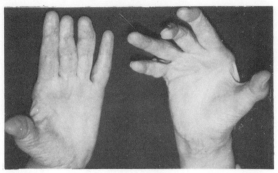

a

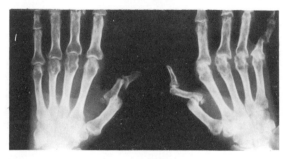

b

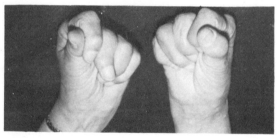

c

Figure 12.35 (a) Swan neck deformity of thumb. (b) X-ray shows gross hyperextension of metacarpophalangeal joint has led to dislocation. (c) Despite considerable joint damage, a remarkable degree of function is maintained

flexor crease and the next (Bruner, 1967). Care must be taken at the angles not to damage the digital nerve. In the palm, incisions should run parallel to but not in joint creases; it is thus easier to evert edges and to avoid maceration from entrapped sweat which lodges in the crease.

(2) To the metacarpophalangeal joint. Incisions may be longitudinal or transverse. The former should be Z-shaped, for it is sometimes necessary to divide the intrinsics. The advantage of this incision is that it is easier to preserve veins and lymphatics, thus reducing the likelihood of post-operative swelling. This is also diminished by meticulous haemostasis, by compression bandaging and post-operative elevation of the limb.

(3) To the proximal interphalangeal joint. For synovectomy a dorso-ulnar approach is required, and for joint replacement an ulnar collateral incision with division of the ulnar ligament.

In operations on the first carpometacarpal joint, care must be taken not to sever the radial nerve or the radial artery and its branch to the thumb.

CONCLUSION

A good deal of surgical aid is available for the rheumatoid hand. It must be stressed, however, that selection of surgical procedures can only be carried out successfully after careful assessment. Good records are indispensable; otherwise the surgeon can be deceived by 'impressions' as to the success of his surgery. It should always be remembered that much help can be provided for the rheumatoid hand by provision of mechanical aids to daily living; surgery should only be carried out when there is a clear indication that the outcome will improve function.

REFERENCES

Benjamin, A. (1976). Double osteotomy for arthritis of the knee, shoulder and finger joints. Clinical demonstration. *6th Combined Meeting. Orth. Ass. Eng. Speaking World*, London

Bruner, J. M. (1967). Zig-zag volar digital incisions for flexor tendon surgery, *Proceedings*

Hand Society 23rd Meeting, 423

Curtis, R. M. (1969). Management of the stiff proximal interphalangeal joint. *Hand*, 1 (1), 32

Flatt, A. E. (1963). *The Cure of the Rheumatoid Hand*, Mosby, St. Louis

Harrison, S. H. and Nicolle, F. V. (1974). A new intramedullary bone peg for digital arthrodesis. *Br. J. Plast. Surg.*, **27**, 240–241

Helal, B. (1967). The silicones as applied to the hand. *J. Br. Club Surg. Hand*, November, 33

Helal, B. (1969). Silicones in orthopaedic surgery. *Recent Advances in Orthopaedics*, Churchill, London

Helal, B. (1970). Distal profundus entrapment in rheumatoid disease. *Hand*, **2** (1), 48

Helal, B. (1974). Proximal interphalangeal joint stiffness in rheumatoid arthritis. *Scand. J. Rheum.*, **3**, 59–62

Kessler, I. (1973). Silicone arthroplasty of the trapezio-metacarpal joint. *J. Bone Jt Surg.*, **55B**, 285–291

Littler, J. W. (1964). Principles of reconstructive surgery of the hand. *Reconstruct. Plast. Surg.*, **4**, 1612

Matev, I. (1964). Transposition of the lateral slips of the aponeurosis in treatment of long-standing 'boutonnière deformity' of the fingers. *Br. J. Plast. Surg.*, **17**, 281

Nicolle, F. V. and Calnan, J. S. (1972). A new design of finger joint prostheses for the rheumatoid hand. *Hand*, **4** (2), 135

Swanson, A. B. (1972). Flexible implant, resection arthroplasty. *Hand*, **4** (2), 119

13

THE HIP JOINT

Rheumatoid disease in the hip causes pain, limitation of movement and deformity. There is osteoporosis, loss of joint space and erosions which may progress to collapse of the upper quadrant of the femoral head with destruction of the upper lip or floor of the acetabulum, producing femoral head subluxation on to the ilium, or central protrusion (figure 13.1). Osteoporosis and bony collapse are aggravated by systemic corticosteroid therapy (figure 13.2). The rheumatoid hip loses movement early, in contradistinction to the rheumatoid knee. Apart from its weight-bearing function, for which stability is required, hip mobility in rheumatoid disease is important, as a stiff hip throws undue strain on other joints during active life and later increases nursing difficulties should the patient become chairbound.

DIAGNOSIS

Characteristically the pain begins in the groin and extends down the inner side of the thigh towards the knee; indeed knee pain may be the presenting symptom. Pain occurs on weight-bearing and at night, the night pain being aggravated by overactivity during the preceding day. One early symptom is difficulty in cutting the toe nails; this complaint may localise the source of pain arising in the hip as distinct from that referred from the spine. Radiologically, rheumatoid disease of the hip is characterised by a uniform diminution of joint-space, whereas in degenerative arthritis the disease tends to affect one or other segment more severely.

TREATMENT

Before considering surgery, every effort is made to relieve pain by conservative measures. If the hip is painless, surgery is seldom indicated. Painless deformity and loss of movement may be an indication for surgery in ankylosing spondylitis. Heat and gentle non-weight-bearing exercises in slings or in a pool may relieve pain and spasm and diminish the rate of destruction of the joint. An electric heat-pad for use at home may give comfort. A walking-stick in the contralateral hand, walking on grass, and wearing shoes with the

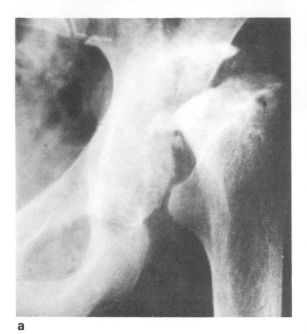
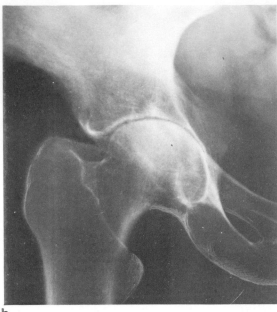

a   b

Figure 13.1 (a) Destruction and subluxation of the femoral head on to the ilium (G. Arden); (b) central protusion (G. Arden)

entire heel thickness made of resilient material will protect both the hips and knees from the repeated impacts which accompany walking. If the foot is held in equinus owing to hip flexion contracture, a raised shoe may relieve pain, although it encourages further deformity.

Flexion contracture may be prevented or reduced by periods of lying prone, by avoiding pillows beneath the knees when in bed, and long uninterrupted periods of sitting.

Non-surgical hospital treatment

In 1956, when rheumatoid hip arthritis was an indication for intertrochanteric osteotomy, a series of cases was treated at West Herts Hospital as for an osteotomy but without being subjected to operation (Rhys Davies and Benjamin, 1962). The patient was admitted, skin traction was applied to the lower limb for 3 weeks, and after discharge from hospital non-weight-bearing with crutches was maintained for 3 months. Half of the patients were completely relieved of pain for 1 year and this relief has so far been maintained in a few patients. There is a place for this treatment if surgery is contra-indicated or has to be delayed.

Local injection of steroids into the hip does not offer lasting benefit and is not advised, in view of the danger of increasing joint destruction, either by the Charcot (neuropathic) effect or by the introduction of infection (Sweetnam, Mason and Murray, 1960).

Surgical treatment

Synovectomy

Synovectomy is beneficial in the early stages of rheumatoid disease of the hip when there is pain without bone destruction. A limited anterior procedure is sufficient and dislocation is unnecessary. Decompression of the joint without synovectomy may be sufficient, as it is the increased intra-articular pressure which impairs the blood supply to the head of the femur, hastening its destruction. Owing to its blood supply, the femoral head in the child is more susceptible to increased intra-articular pressure . than in the adult. Usually the disease is too advanced for synovectomy by the time the orthopaedic surgeon is consulted.

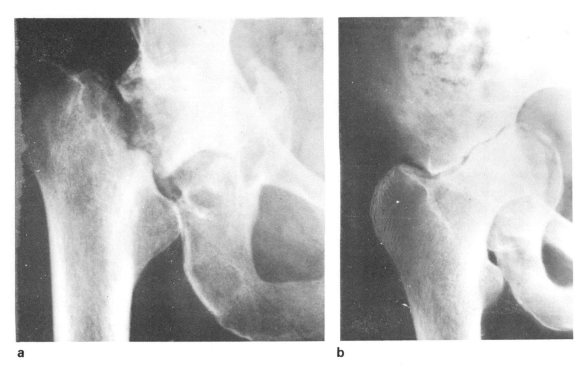

Figure 13.2 Bony collapse aggravated by systemic corticosteroid therapy; (a) spontaneous Girdlestone; (b) central dislocation

Adductor tenotomy

Tenotomy of the hip adductor muscles adjacent to the lesser trochanter is a useful adjunct to other operative procedures, but is seldom of value on its own. This tenotomy may, for example, allow abduction after a Girdlestone excision arthroplasty. It is seldom indicated in total hip replacement, as a fixed adduction deformity usually corrects spontaneously in the 6 months following total replacement.

Psoas tenotomy

Tenotomy of the psoas tendon adjacent to its insertion on the lesser trochanter, through a small posterior skin incision often relieves hip pain associated with muscle spasm. It seldom gives lasting benefit but may provide several months of relief for an elderly patient unfit for major surgery.

Osteotomy

Intertrochanteric osteotomy for pain in rheumatoid disease is not as rewarding as in degenerative arthritis and it has been suggested there

is no place for it in rheumatoid disease, owing to occasional post-operative collapse of the femoral head. We believe that osteotomy has a valuable but limited place. It is indicated when total replacement is inadvisable, for example, in the presence of varicose ulceration, severe psoriasis and where degenerative arthritis is superimposed on a hip in which the rheumatoid process is quiescent.

Technique

The patient is placed supine on the operating table with a small pad under the buttock of the affected side. Draping allows the leg to be manipulated during the operation. The incision is longitudinal, 25 mm (1 inch) in front of the mid-lateral line extending from 25 mm (1 inch) proximal to the tip of the great trochanter to 150 mm (6 inches) distal to it. The slightly anterior incision gives a good view of the anterior aspect of the femur and facilitates the positioning of the medial osteotome; some surgeons prefer to operate with the patient on an orthopaedic table and to make a more posterior incision. The great trochanter with the proximal limit of the vastus lateralis muscle and 100 mm (4 inches) of femoral shaft are exposed. The lesser trochanter is palpated medially and two bone levers are inserted, one proximal and one distal. Osteotomy is at the level of the lesser trochanter between these two bone levers and is at right angles to the shaft of the femur, not oblique. If the femur is cut carelessly, a spur of bone from the medial cortex of the distal fragment may extend proximally under the neck of the femur (figure 13.3) and prevent accurate displacement. An accurate osteotomy is made by drilling 3-mm ($\frac{1}{8}$ inch) holes along the projected line; the medial cortex is then cut with a narrow, vertically placed osteotome and a transversely directed one completes the osteotomy (figure 5.11 and figure 13.4).

The use of a mechanical saw can cause bone necrosis, especially if the blade is blunt, and this may give rise to non-union. A wedge excision is unnecessary, for angulation is easy to obtain without it. Moreover a wedge causes unnecessary shortening and further increases the probability of non-union (figure 5.13). If the hip is mobile, a few degrees of varus displacement may be beneficial. It is important for the surgeon to remain aware of the position of the patella to avoid rotational displacement. Internal fixation with a Wainwright spline (1970) (figure 13.5) is simple and effective; the displacement of the distal fragment medially, necessary to insert the spline, reduces the forces on the hip joint by reducing the horizontal lever arm from the shaft to head (Milch, 1965; Osborne and Fahrni, 1950). This displacement does not interfere significantly with the insertion of a total hip prosthesis should it be indicated at a later date, for bone remodelling usually reforms the medullary canal (see figure 13.26). The spline allows the bone-ends to slide together and close any gap arising from bone necrosis and does not hold them apart as sometimes occurs with more rigid fixation. A compression nail-plate can also increase bone necrosis at the osteotomy site.

Pauwels (1961) has suggested that angulation should be either varus or valgus, depending upon the congruity of the femoral head on X-rays in abduction and adduction taken before operation. His theory is attractive, but we find little evidence that the appropriate correction gives improved clinical results. Varus, valgus and undisplaced

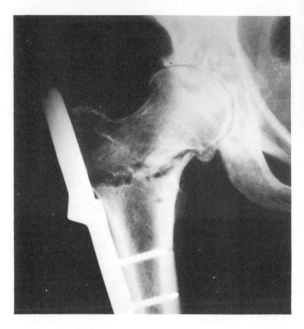

Figure 13.3 A technically poor osteotomy with a spur; the case did well nevertheless. See figure 13.6c

osteotomies appear to be equally satisfactory (figure 13.6).

A successful intertrochanteric osteotomy commonly relieves pain for seven or eight years and often for longer. Clinical improvement is accompanied by X-ray evidence of an increase in joint-space over several years (figure 13.7).

Excision arthroplasty

The Girdlestone (1943) excision arthroplasty has an important place in the treatment of rheumatoid hip disease. This procedure has fallen into disrepute due to lack of attention to detail given in the early post-operative period. After a technically satisfactory Girdlestone procedure the majority of patients will have a pain-free hip with good movement. The disadvantages are some loss of leg length and a Trendelenburg limp due to failure of the relatively lengthened abductor muscles to hold the trunk over the weight-bearing leg.

The indications for excision arthroplasty of the hip are infection of a previous prosthetic replacement, failure of a prosthesis from some other cause or the painful rheumatoid hip, in which both

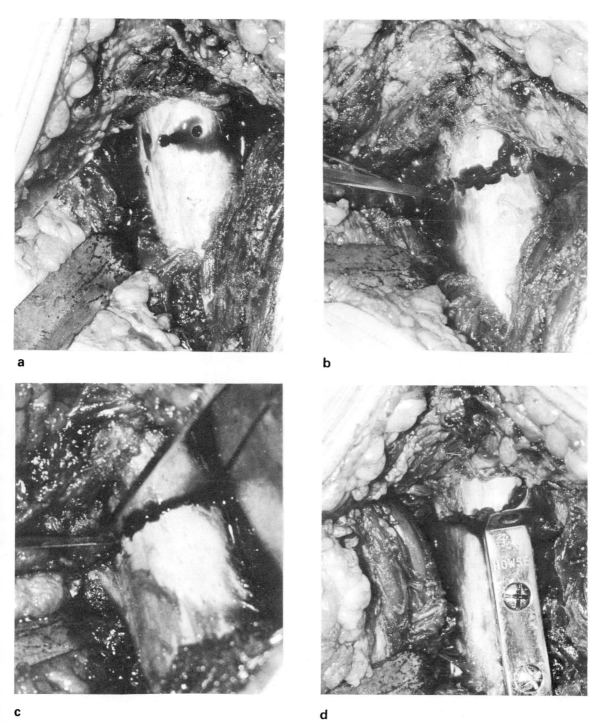

a

b

c

d

Figure 13.4 Intertrochanteric osteotomy. Compare with figure 5.11: (a) 3-mm (⅛ inch) drill-holes; (b) narrow osteotome in medial cortex; (c) broader osteotome from lateral cortex meeting narrow osteotome; (d) internal fixation with a Wainwright spline

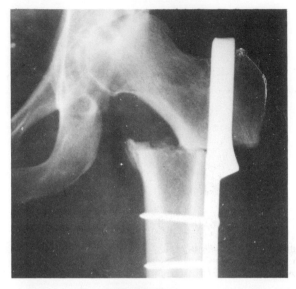

Figure 13.5 Internal fixation with a Wainwright spline. Marked displacement is necessary to achieve varus angulation

prosthetic replacement and osteotomy are contra-indicated. Prosthetic replacement may be contra-indicated by skin disease or resistant varicose ulceration and osteotomy may be contra-indicated by imminent collapse of the femoral head. Although revision of a total hip prosthesis may be justifiable, it should be remembered that the complication rate of revision is high, and it may be officious surgery to persist in replacing prostheses, for the alternative of excision arthroplasty will provide a painless hip with less risk (figures 13.8 and 13.9).

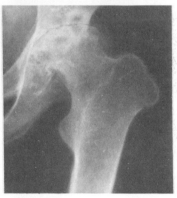
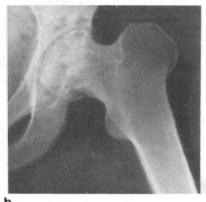
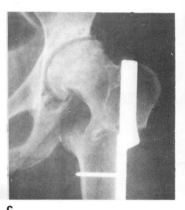

b   c

Figure 13.6 (a) Adduction, poor joint-space, head not contained; (b) hip abducted, better joint-space with congruity, hip contained—should benefit from adduction osteotomy; (c) 1 year after abduction osteotomy, improved joint-space and pain-free

Figure 13.7 Improvements in joint-space following intertrochanteric osteotomy: (a) pre-operative; (b) six months post-operative; (c) 3 years post-operative

a   b   c

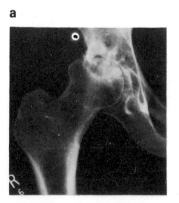
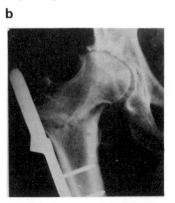
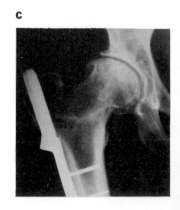

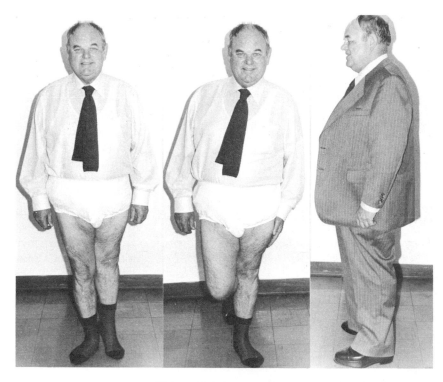

Technique

Through an anterior or anterolateral incision, the head and the neck of the femur are excised at the base of the neck. Excision of the upper lip of the acetabulum, the importance of which has been emphasised in the past, is unnecessary (Haw and Gray, 1976). The lower limb is then abducted and the degree of abduction carefully assessed by palpating the anterior iliac spines. It is essential that the hip can be abducted passively at least 10 —if necessary, with the help of an adductor tenotomy. After skin closure a Steinmann pin is inserted through the upper tibia, and traction [3.2 kg (7 lb)] is applied in the ward to maintain abduction. To prevent the pelvis from rotating, the contralateral lower limb is also abducted (figure 13.10). The skeletal traction has very little, if any, effect either on the leg length or on the space between the upper end of the femur and the pelvis. There is surprisingly little tendency for the shortening to increase and particularly so when the Girdlestone procedure follows prosthetic hip replacement. Neutral rotation of the lower limb is maintained by 0.25 kg ($\frac{1}{2}$ lb) traction applied vertically at one end of the Steinmann pin, or, if

Figure 13.8 Fourteen years after a left Girdlestone excision arthroplasty. The left lower limb is short, the patient can stand on his left foot and his limbs are cosmetically acceptable with a raise on his shoe

Figure 13.9 X-ray of patient shown in figure 13.8

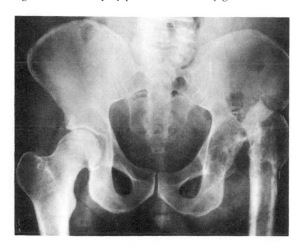

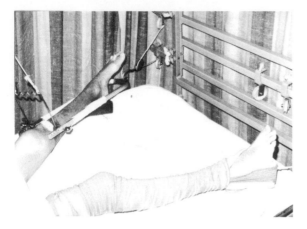

Figure 13.10 Traction on both lower limbs to prevent pelvic rotation and so maintain abduction

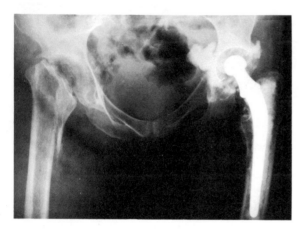

Figure 13.11 Girdlestone operation after a failed total replacement. Notice the few degrees of abduction of the hip.

necessary, by a leg plaster with an anti-rotation bar. The maintenance of abduction and neutral rotation will determine the result of this procedure.

When excision arthroplasty follows removal of a total hip prosthesis, stability due to periarticular fibrosis is such that 6 weeks' immobilisation on traction is adequate, whereas if this is a primary surgical procedure, it is desirable to maintain traction in abduction and neutral rotation for 12 weeks (figure 13.11). Daily supervision of the traction and meticulous care in maintaining the position are essential. Failure to maintain abduction will result in a fixed adduction deformity with an increase in apparent shortening and a shearing stress across the pseudarthrosis, with less stability and more pain. Stability and relief of pain may be restored by an abduction osteotomy (figure 13.12).

Interposition arthroplasty

In 1895 Robert Jones interposed gold foil in a pseudarthrosis created in the subtrochanteric region (Jones, 1908). Since then skin and fascia have been used and later a vitallium cup described by Smith-Petersen (1925, 1935). Interposition nylon cups provoke considerable tissue reaction owing to the microscopic particles of nylon from wear of the cup. Interposition arthroplasty of the hip has a limited place, as it has been largely superseded by total prosthetic replacement.

Figure 13.12 Adduction deformity after a Girdlestone operation treated by osteotomy: (a) the deformity; (b) immediately after an abduction osteotomy; (c) 8 years after osteotomy

a   **b**   **c**

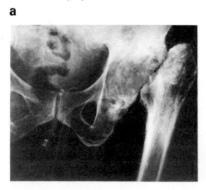
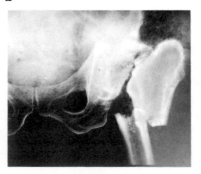
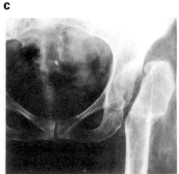

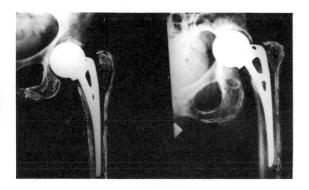

Figure 13.13 A replacement femoral head boring into the porotic bone of the pelvis

Replacement of the femoral head

Femoral head replacements such as Judet, Austin Moore or Thompson are unsuitable, owing to the rheumatoid process affecting the acetabulum. They do not relieve pain and are likely to protrude into the pelvis (figure 13.13).

Total hip replacement

Philip Wiles designed a prosthetic hip joint and replaced several hips in the 1930s. Unfortunately the X-rays and case records were destroyed during the Second World War air raids (Wiles, 1957).

In 1951 McKee at Norwich constructed a total hip prosthesis of stainless steel. As this was unsuccessful, he changed the material to cobalt – chrome alloy and utilised acrylic cement described by Haboush in 1953 (McKee and Watson Farrar, 1966); the femoral component was based on the Thompson femoral head and stem and was cemented into the femoral shaft. The acetabular cup was constructed with protruding studs to improve keying into the cement with which it was held in the acetabulum. This prosthesis has proved successful and has stood the test of time.

John Charnley (1959) reported on the lubrication of animal joints and he produced a prosthesis consisting of a high-density polythene RCH 100 cup and a femoral component of 18–8 molybdenum stainless steel. These were cemented into the acetabulum and femoral shaft with self-curing acrylic resin. By the use of stainless steel on high-density polythene and a small femoral head, Charnley reduced the friction between the two

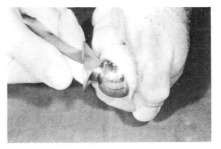

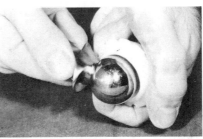

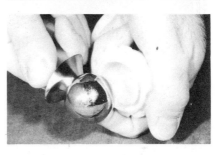

Figure 13.14 The Howse snap-on hip prosthesis. The prosthesis can only be taken apart by levering the neck on the rim of the cup (D. Howse and Co.)

components, thus diminishing the strain at the cement – bone interface.

Many designs of metal on plastics prostheses are now on the market. We have used the Charnley, the McKee and the Howse prostheses; in one design of the latter the femoral head snaps into the acetabulum, thus decreasing the risk of dislocation (figure 13.14).

Owing to the disadvantages of cement, Ring (1968) developed a total hip prosthesis of cobalt – chromium alloy which does not require cement. The femoral head has a stem of Austin Moore type and the cup a long threaded stem for pelvic fixation (figure 13.15). Considerable skill is required to insert this prosthesis accurately.

The introduction of the total hip prosthesis by McKee has done as much to relieve human

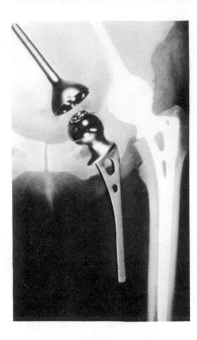

Figure 13.15 The Ring prosthesis

suffering as any other recent surgical development. Charnley's use of the low-friction properties of metal on plastics is the most significant improvement and most new prostheses will incorporate the low-friction, principle. Of new materials being tried, ceramics possess useful properties but are not yet acceptable for general use (Boutin, 1972). New non-cemented prostheses with porous external surfaces into which bone can grow are under trial.

Integral total prostheses in which the acetabulum and head of femur are inserted as a single unit are recommended for the treatment of subcapital femoral fractures (figure 13.16a). They may be of value in the older rheumatoid patient, as the operation is technically simple and no cement is necessary.

The double cup design now at an early stage in development shows promise (figure 13.16b).

Several hundred different designs of hip prostheses are now available and it is tempting to experiment if they have some feature which seems advantageous. We believe it is better for the surgeon to become adept in the use of one design and not to change, provided his results are satisfactory.

Indications

Severe pain, not responding to conservative measures is the main indication for total prosthetic replacement of the rheumatoid hip. Pain severity is assessed by the analgesic requirement, the consequent impairment of function and loss of sleep. If a Girdlestone operation is preferable to the patient's current situation, then there is unequivocal indication for total hip replacement.

Pre-operative considerations

Age It is best to avoid total hip replacement in the young active individual; however, in patients whose activity is already restricted by general rheumatoid disease the lower age limit is reduced and may include children with juvenile polyarthritis (Ansell and Arden, 1979). There is no upper age limit and an expectation of life over 6 months may well justify this operation, which dramatically reduces pain and requires such a short period of rehabilitation.

Which first, hip or knee? Fixed flexion deformity of a knee of 30° or more interferes with the recovery of an ipsilateral total hip prosthesis, as it predisposes to dislocation of the hip. On the other hand, abduction or adduction deformity of the hip throws a strain on a total knee prosthesis which may seriously interfere with its function (figure 13.17). Opinions differ, but when both hip and knee require surgery, it is generally better to operate on the 'worse' first or to do both, with a short interval between, only allowing the patient to walk after both joints have been replaced.

Bilateral replacement When both hips require surgery, total replacements can be performed simultaneously. However, this engenders undue morbidity and we prefer to operate on each hip separately, with an interval of 1–3 months.

Steroids Systemic steroid therapy causes decalcification and consequently increases the likelihood of failure at the cement–bone interface; it also increases the probability of deep infection. If long-term steroid therapy has been introduced, it is

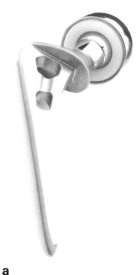

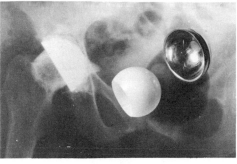

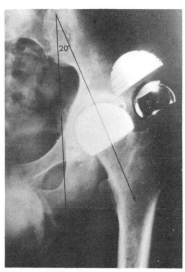

b

Figure 13.16 (a) A hard-top Monk integral hip prosthesis (D. Howse and Co.); (b) the ICLH double cup preliminary model; (c) the materials have since been reversed to a plastic acetabular and a metal capital component (M. Freeman)

a

c

preferable for it to be discontinued or reduced sometime before surgery.

Infection A successful total hip replacement, in a patient severely disabled by pain, is little short of a miracle, but the total hip replacement which develops deep infection is a major catastrophe. The possibility of infection has to be discussed with the patient, before operation, and both surgeon and patient must consider the risk justifiable. Most authorities agree that deep infection is more likely to occur in rheumatoid disease than in degenerative arthritis. Certain standards of simple hygiene favour a lower infection rate and the mere change from an old to a new operating theatre suite with no alteration in staffing or technique has effected a reduction in cases of deep infection. The incidence of deep infection may be reduced by careful attention to details (table 6.1, p. 68).

Pre-operative assessment The pre-operative general examination often reveals symptoms and signs of cardiovascular, respiratory, skin or other disease. Any such problems should be fully investigated and treated by the appropriate medical or surgical department before operation. Catheterisation following total hip replacement is undesirable (chapter 6), and if indications of incipient prostatic obstruction exist, this should be relieved surgically in advance.

Figure 13.17 The valgus knee requires total replacement but the hip is fixed in adduction and must be replaced first

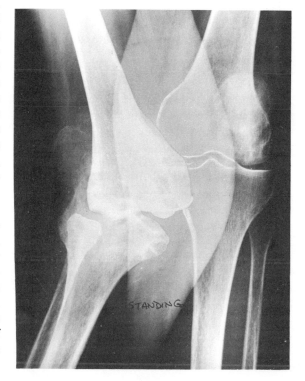

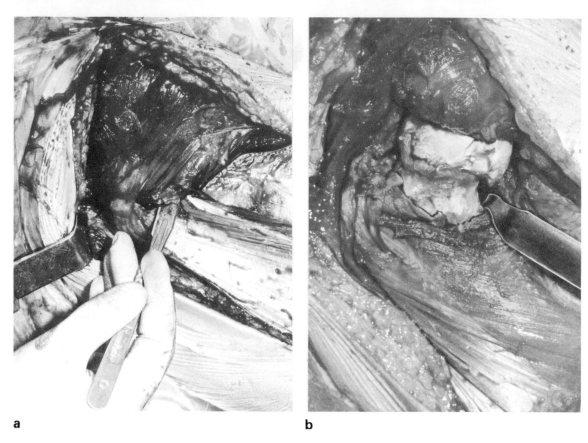

a   b

Figure 13.18   Anterolateral approach to the hip joint. The anterior 25 mm (1 inch) of the insertion of gluteus medius is cut, (a) enabling the hip to be exposed and dislocated, (b) without removal of the trochanter

Operative technique

John Charnley approaches the hip joint through a lateral incision with the patient lying supine. He detaches the great trochanter and, when closing, he advocates reattaching it, a little more distally, to improve the mechanical advantage of the hip abductor muscles. We feel that the routine removal of the great trochanter is unnecessary, but that an approach similar to that of Charnley or a posterior approach gives adequate exposure in most cases. If it does not, then at any time during the operation the great trochanter may be removed to improve access. In order to ream the acetabulum, Charnley drills a hole into the pelvis from the floor of the acetabulum and his expanding reamer is centred into this hole. We feel that, as a routine measure, this hole adds unnecessary complications, for it weakens the acetabular floor and requires the insertion of a cement restricter; it may

allow infection to pass from the pelvis to the joint, and if cement enters the pelvis through the hole, considerable difficulty may be encountered should it need removing later. The acetabulum can be reamed adequately without the centring hole using standard gouges and reamers or the Charnley expanding reamer with the centring knob removed.

Anterolateral approach without removing the trochanter The patient is placed supine and draped, leaving the lower limb free to be manipulated during the operation. The incision is 205 mm (8 inches) long, centred over the tip of the great trochanter, the distal half parallel with the femur and the proximal directed a few degrees posteriorly. The space between the tensor fascia lata and the gluteus medius muscle is developed. The

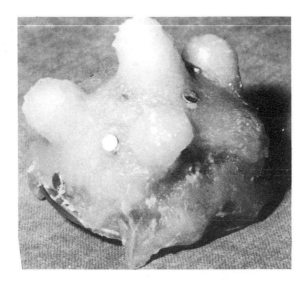

Figure 13.19 A McKee–Farrar cup with its surrounding cement which has been removed because of loosening. Note the casts of the keying holes in cement, intended to prevent loosening. (G. Arden)

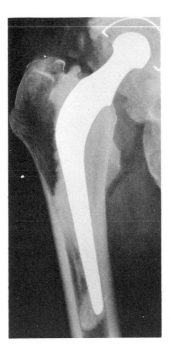

Figure 13.20 The cement has not entered the great trochanter because cancellous bone is preventing it. It is better to gouge out some of the cancellous tissue to allow the cement to key against cortical bone

anterior 25 mm (1 inch) of the attachment of the gluteus medius to the great trochanter is divided (figure 13.18). Care is taken when dislocating the hip to do so with skids in the joint and to use little or no leverage on the femoral shaft, which, weakened by rheumatoid disease and perhaps corticosteroids, is liable to fracture. The technique proceeds along the lines described by Charnley, except that the centring hole penetrating the pelvic cavity is omitted and consequently different reaming instruments are used. In rheumatoid disease it is seldom necessary to deepen the acetabulum, but removal of cartilage and other soft tissue is recommended, as also is the drilling of keying holes into the ilium, the ischium and the pubis (figure 13.19). The cancellous bone should be removed from within the great trochanter to ensure that the cement keys to the stronger cortical bone (figure 13.20). The preparation of the femoral shaft with the femoral broach is undertaken entirely by hand, as the injudicious use of a mallet increases the likelihood of piercing the cortex or shattering the femoral neck. The insertion of the femoral component may be impeded by bony resistance which is not relieved by further medullary reaming. This resistance may be

due to obstruction of the shoulder of the prosthesis at the femoral neck and trochanter. The routine use of a rectangular box chisel before broaching and reaming the femoral shaft eliminates this problem (figure 13.21). It is the relative position of cup to head that determines the ultimate stability of the hip. It is important to ensure that the femoral head is pointing directly into the centre of the cup, that is, neither ante- nor retroverted when the lower limb lies in the position of rest.

During the operation the limb is manipulated to dislocate the femoral head and to expose the acetabulum and femoral neck for their preparation. Care is necessary, on the part of the assistant, to avoid undue strain on the knee, which may also be arthritic. Flexion beyond 90° is best avoided.

Posterior approach The posterior approach enables the prosthesis to be inserted with less difficulty but may increase the risks of infection and

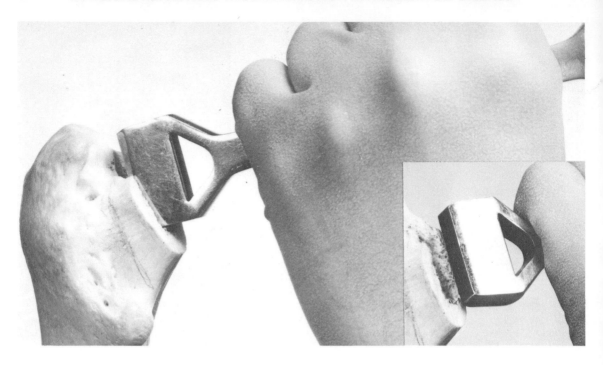

Figure 13.21 The rectangular box chisel (D. Howse and Co.)

dislocation. Despite these possible disadvantages many surgeons prefer this approach.

The anaesthetised patient lies on the contralateral side and is draped such that the affected limb may be manipulated during the operation. The incision, 254 mm (10 inches) in length, is centred on the great trochanter, the distal limb is parallel to the shaft of the femur and the proximal curves gently towards the posterior superior iliac spine. Subcutaneous tissue and deep fascia are divided in the line of the incision, over the great trochanter. The limb is then lifted by an assistant, relaxing the deep fascia, which is slit in the line of the incision in both directions with scissors. The gluteal fascia is incised in the line of the incision and the hip is internally rotated. The posterior border of the glutei and distal to that the upper border of the quadratus femoris can be seen separated by fat. Dissection through this exposes the tendons of the obturator internus and the two gemelli. At this stage the position of the sciatic nerve is ascertained; it is usually easy to palpate. Fat and fascia are dissected from the obturator and gemelli tendons by blunt dissection with a swab. A stout stay suture is inserted into these tendons and, with the hip well internally rotated, the three tendons are cut, exposing, but not penetrating the capsule of the hip joint. The pyriformis muscle occasionally extends over the joint and needs to be cut with the obturator and gemelli. The short rotators are swung back over the sciatic nerve, retracted with the stay suture. Some fibres of glutei arise from the capsule, in line with the neck, and it is helpful to cut the edge of these fibres to allow a bone-lever to pass between them and the capsule. Two Bristow-type bone-levers are placed one above and one below the neck of the femur and a cruciate incision is made into the capsule. The bone-levers are now transferred within the capsule above and below the neck, and by internally rotating the hip and perhaps flexing, it is dislocated with the help of a skid. The acetabulum and the femur are prepared and the prosthesis inserted. If possible, the capsule is sutured, and it is advisable to repair the rotator muscles, fixing them back firmly to the trochanter, using an awl to make a hole for the stay suture, thus holding the rotator tendons well down to bone. Some surgeons do not consider it necessary to repair these muscles.

Total hip replacement with an absent or weak acetabular floor Central dislocation of the acetabular component may be prevented by:

(1) Using the femoral head as a bone graft for the floor of the acetabulum.

(2) Using a vitallium mesh.

(3) Using an Eichler ring.

(4) Using a combination of vitallium mesh and Eichler ring.

(5) Using a prosthetic cup with a flange.

(6) Using a specially made deep acetabular cup.

The femoral head can be cut into thin slices and used as a graft to strengthen the floor of the acetabulum. The slices are placed to strengthen the thin or absent acetabular floor but to avoid those areas, including the acetabular roof, which give stability and keying for cement. The cement is inserted when it is of such a consistency that it will not flow between the slices of graft, or between the graft and the prepared acetabular floor (figure 13.22).

Figure 13.22 Grafting of the acetabular floor for protusio; (a) and (b) slicing of the femoral head; (c) preop; (d) graft incorporated in the acetabular floor

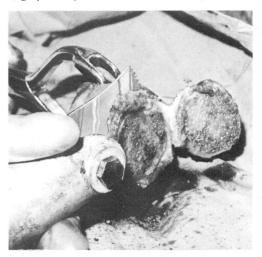

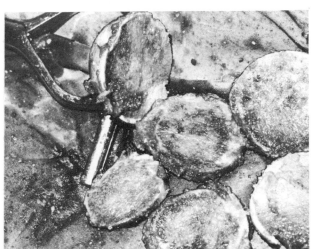

a

b

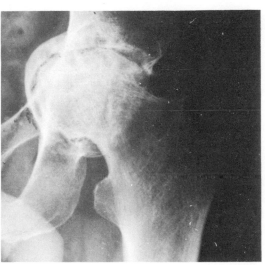

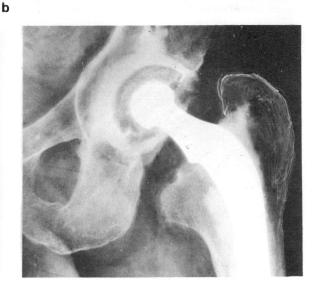

c

d

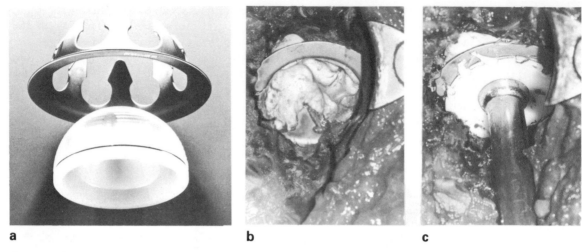

a   b   c

Figure 13.23 The Eichler ring: (a) the ring and a cup (Synthes); (b) the ring inserted with freshly mixed cement in it; (c) The cup has been inserted and is being held firmly in place while the cement sets

The Eichler ring is good support but may be further strengthened by vitallium mesh. The principle of the Eichler ring, and of the large flanged cup, is to rely upon the rim of the acetabulum rather than its floor for resisting central dislocation. After preparation of the acetabulum, the supporting Eichler ring is provisionally placed in position. It must rest with its flange resting directly on the entire circumference of the acetabular lip. Three notches are cut into the rim of the acetabulum to act as cement-keying holes. Cement is placed deep to the Eichler ring and between the ring and the prosthesis, which are held firmly in their desired position while the cement is setting. The technique is not easy and should be attempted only by surgeons already proficient in hip replacement surgery (Eichler, 1973; Schatzker and Hastings, 1976; figures 13.23–13.24).

Arden has designed a prosthetic cup with a 5 mm ($\frac{1}{4}$ inch) flange as an intrinsic part of its design (figure 13.25). This redistributes weight-bearing to the acetabular rim without the complication of an additional prosthesis.

Total hip replacement after intertrochanteric osteotomy Removal of internal fixation apparatus at the same time as the insertion of a prosthetic total hip replacement is inadvisable, as the likelihood of complications is increased. The plate or spline and screws from the internal fixation of the inter-

trochanteric osteotomy should be removed at least 3 months before the hip replacement. During this time the damage to both bone and soft tissues recovers. Owing to bone remodelling and the reformation of the medullary canal, there is usually no difficulty in inserting the femoral stem, despite displacement at the osteotomy site (figure 13.26). If required, the medullary cavity may be accurately drilled with the help of a simple jig

Figure 13.24 Total hip replacement with Eichler ring

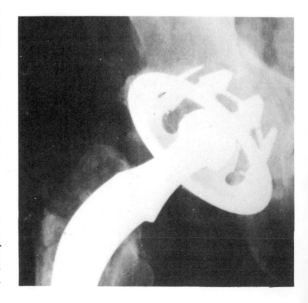

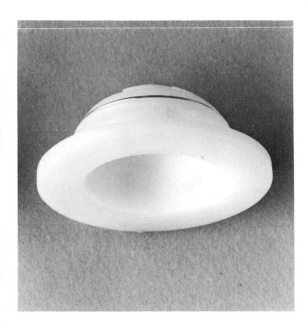

Figure 13.25 The Arden flanged cup made by Zimmer

designed by Read (figure 13.27). A more complicated jig has been designed by Charnley.

Total prosthesis following bony fusion of hip Bony fusion of the hip due to ankylosis or to an arthrodesis may be treated by total replacement arthroplasty, even after many years, and results in a useful mobile hip (Hardinge *et al.*, 1977). The indications are: deformity of the fused hip, causing strain on the spine, and multiple joint disease, in which a stiff hip compounds the disability. The head and neck of the femur are exposed through an anterolateral incision, the neck is sectioned and the acetabular cavity is reamed. The operation then proceeds along routine lines (figure 13.28).

Complications

Dislocation Dislocation may occur when moving from the operating table to the recovery room and the ward. The hip is stable in internal rotation following the anterolateral approach and in external rotation and extension following the posterior approach; for both approaches it is stable in abduction. If there is doubt about the stability, an abduction wedge is advisable until the sutures are removed 2 weeks post-operatively. Following the anterolateral approach, the hip may be safeguard-

Fig 13.26 Reformation of the medullary canal by bone remodelling after osteotomy: (a) immediately after operation; (b) 4 months post-operative; (c) 3 years post-operative

a

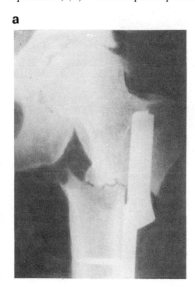

b

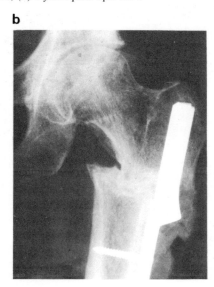

c

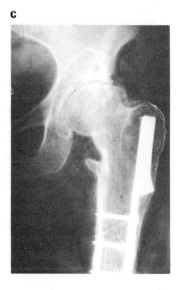

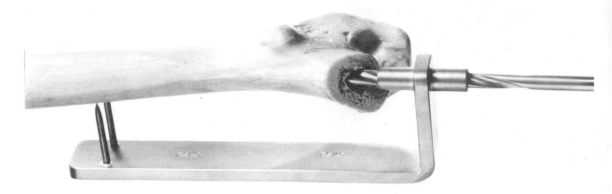

Figure 13.27 The Read jig, which enables a drill to be accurately directed along the medullary canal (D. Howse and Co.)

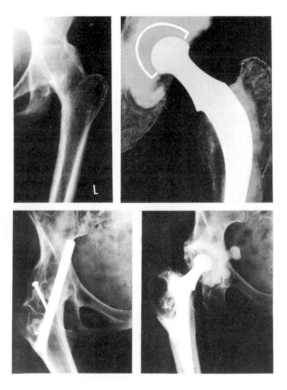

Figure 13.28 Two cases of arthrodesed hips which have been replaced by prostheses. Back ache was relieved, apparent shortening was corrected and a surprising degree of control of the hip muscles ensued in spite of the hips having been fixed, one for 9 years and the other for 15 years

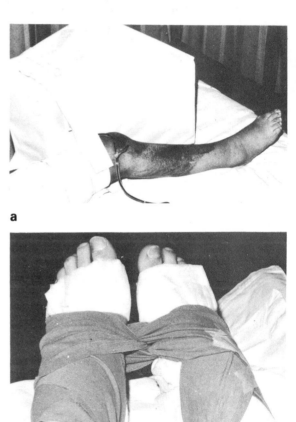

a

b

Figure 13.29 Prevention of dislocation immediately after total replacement: (a) abduction wedge; (b) the feet bandaged together to prevent external rotation

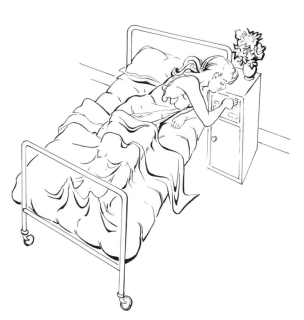

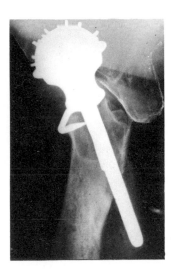

Figure 13.31 Projection of the femoral stem through the posterior cortex

Figure 13.30 The bedside locker encourages internal rotation of the hip nearest to it and external rotation of the other

ed by bandaging the two feet together, thus preventing external rotation, until the patient is awake in the ward. Orthopaedic wool between the feet and ankles prevents pressure sores (figure 13.29). Following the posterior approach, the patient is not allowed to sit in a chair or in bed until the sutures are removed, but during that time is allowed both to lie down or stand, thus maintaining extension of the hip. After an anterior approach, the patient's bedside locker should be placed on the same side as the operated hip, as turning to it will rotate the hip medially, whereas after a posterior approach, the locker is placed on the other side, as turning to it will externally rotate the hip (figure 13.30).

After discharge from hospital, the patient is advised to avoid crossing the legs and sitting low for several weeks. Seat raises are available for low toilets.

Should dislocation occur, closed reduction under general anaesthetic is generally possible, and if abduction is maintained for 3 weeks, the hip usually becomes stable. It is possible, by means of a cast-brace with a pelvic band holding the hip in abduction, to mobilise the patient with an unstable hip. If dislocation recurs or stability cannot be maintained, revision or conversion to a Girdlestone excision arthroplasty is indicated.

Incorrect reaming of the femur The posterior cortex of the femoral shaft may be pierced by misdirecting the reamer or broach (figure 13.31). This complication is less likely with the posterior approach or if the trochanter is removed in the anterolateral approach. When the shaft is narrow and difficult to ream, the posterior cortex may be damaged, even in experienced hands. In order to avoid this, the direction of the shaft should be clearly visualised and the reamer directed along it. If the thigh lies parallel to the operating table, then the reamer also must be parallel to it. In the anterolateral approach this is facilitated by the skin incision being curved posteriorly in its proximal third. Reaming and broaching should be undertaken by hand rather than with the broach and hammer to avoid posterior cortical damage and shattering of the femoral neck.

Fracture of the femur Spiral fractures of the femoral shaft may occur in the proximity of the femoral prosthesis either at operation, or at any time post-operatively due to trauma. Replacement by a long-stemmed femoral prosthesis is a major

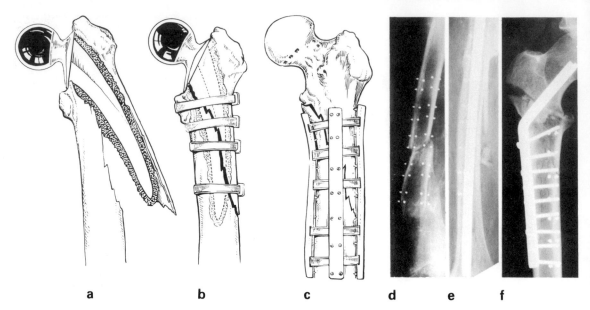

| a | b | c | d | e | f |

Figure 13.32 Chichester straps and plates for the internal fixation of femoral fractures (a & b) a fracture about a prosthesis stem; (c) an oblique fracture; (d) X-ray of transverse fracture (straps and plates); (e) X-ray of comminuted fracture (straps, plates and intramedullary nail); (f) X-ray of intertrochanteric fracture with comminution of shaft (straps, plates and nail plate)

and tedious operation especially if cement has to be removed (chapter 6). More conservative treatment, however, will often result in union without femoral component loosening. In an attempt to eliminate long immobilisation in bed, plates and straps are being developed to fix these fractures internally. The straps are made of Nylon 66 and when tightened will not come undone; they have bumps on the inner side which prevent strangulation of the periosteal blood supply. The straps may be used on their own (Partridge, 1976: see also chapters 1 and 6) or in association with slotted, metal-studded nylon plates (Partridge, 1977; figures 13.32 and 1.8). These Chichester plates and straps are being modified and when released for general use are likely to have valuable applications.

Thrombophlebitis Deep vein thrombosis may occur during the first 2 weeks following total hip replacement. Opinions differ as to its prevention and management; low doses of heparin given pre- and post-operatively are recommended by some authorities (Lowe *et al.*, 1976); prophylactic warfarin or aspirin by others; intermittent calf pressure applied by pneumatic cuffs may help, but

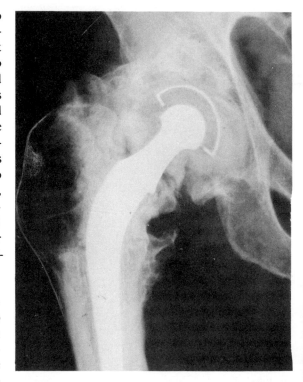

Figure 13.33 Ectopic calcification following total hip replacement

firm bandaging, from the toes to above the knee, for the period of confinement to bed may be sufficient.

Infection This has been dealt with in chapter 6. Deep infection within a sinus can rarely be cured but it may be worth while excising the sinus and dripping a bactericidal agent such as noxythiolin through a tube, inserted down to the prosthesis, and applying suction through another, for 3–4 weeks. If this fails and there is pain, remove the prosthesis and cement immediately rather than spend months or even years giving antibiotics and hoping the infection will 'go away'. Occasionally low-grade infection, with minimal discharge and a painless hip, is acceptable in an elderly patient and sacrifice of the prosthesis is not indicated.

Ectopic calcification Following total hip replacement, excessive calcium can be deposited in the soft tissues around the joint (Brooker *et al.*, 1973; figure 13.33). This ectopic calcification is associated with pain which usually resolves as the hip ankyloses spontaneously. Revision is seldom successful, owing to recurrence of the calcification, and prosthetic replacement of the contralateral hip is likely to suffer the same fate. Di- and polyphosphonates have been used experimentally to prevent this ectopic deposition but their value is not yet established (Bigvoet *et al.*, 1974; Russell, 1975).

Loosening (chapter 6) Loosening of one or both of the components may occur, due to technical failure, infection or metal sensitivity. The patient often complains of pain and a sharp groin pain on heel percussion is a useful sign. The cause must be ascertained to manage the problem correctly. Loosening may be obvious, with one of the components moving on either routine or stress X-ray (figure 13.34), or it may be suggested by a radiolucent zone developing between the cement and bone or between the cement and prosthesis (figure 13.35). This latter appearance may be present for many years, during which the hip is painless and is functioning well. It is not known whether the clear zone on X-ray, in the otherwise normal patient, is an indication of inevitable

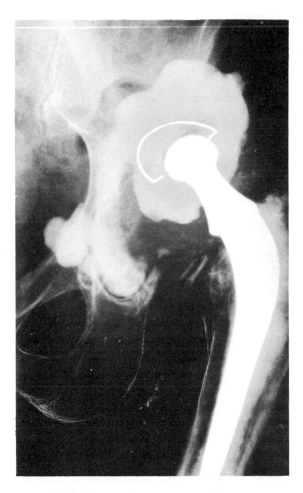

Figure 13.34 Obvious loosening of the cup and much of its surrounding cement

loosening, but such a hip frequently functions efficiently until the patient's death from natural causes. Periostitis of the lateral femoral cortex at the level of the tip of the stem is also an indication of loosening.

If loosening is thought to be the cause of pain, the hip may be X-ray screened, although this is seldom diagnostic, whereas an arthrogram in which the dye tracks between the cement and bone may be diagnostic; however, even this sign may be present in a hip free from symptoms (figure 13.36).

Fracture of the femoral stem Stress fracture of the femoral stem in its middle third and curiously near the tip is not uncommon (figure 13.37). This

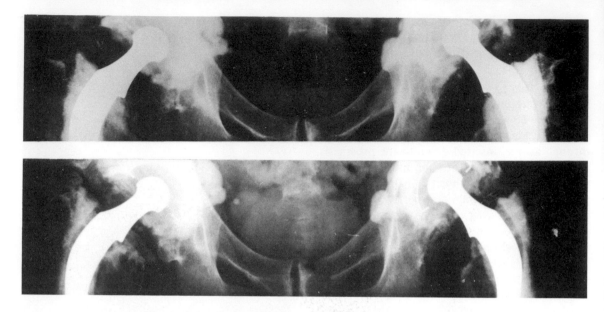

Figure 13.35 X-rays taken 1 year (top) and 5 years (bottom) after bilateral total hip replacement. The clear zone is seen developing between the cement and the prosthesis. In this patient it is symptom-free and there are no other indications of loosening

occurs usually after the fourth post-operative year and in patients weighing over 80 kg (175 lb). Inadequate fixation in the femoral shaft may pre-dispose to fracture. Removal of cancellous bone in the trochanter and packing this space with cement improves the fixation of the upper third of the prosthesis and reduces stress on the middle third. Charnley advises the use of strengthened femoral components in heavier patients.

Undiagnosed pain The patient who presents with groin pain, and whose total prosthetic hip has hitherto given several years of pain-free activity, presents an important management problem. Immediate admission to hospital is recommended, and if there is an unavoidable delay, crutches should be used to avoid weight-bearing. Loosening, prosthetic fracture or infection may be the causes, and are appropriately treated. The differential diagnosis is frequently difficult. The erythrocyte sedimentation rate may be elevated without other evidence of infection, and may or may not indicate infection, whereas anti-staphylococcal and antistreptolysin titres are valu-

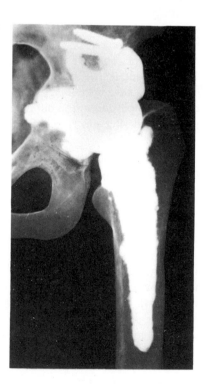

Figure 13.36 Arthrogram with dye tracking around the entire prosthesis (G. Arden)

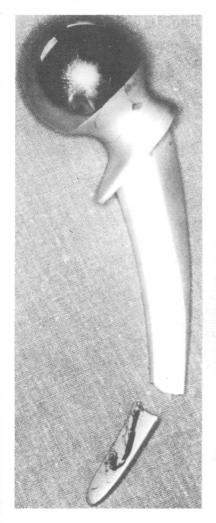 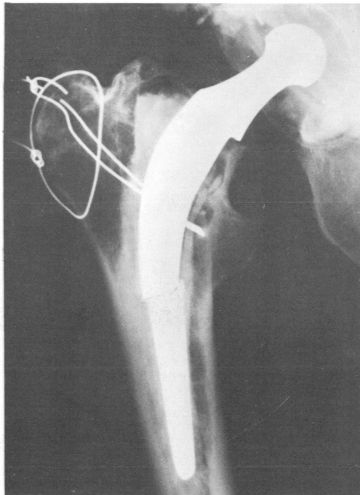

Figure 13.37 Femoral stem fractures

able. If no apparent cause for the pain is revealed, there may be a stress fracture of the acetabulum or of the femur invisible on X-ray. Although the diagnosis is uncertain, the management is not. The patient is confined to bed and 2 kg (5 lb) longitudinal skin traction applied to the leg. This is maintained for 6 weeks, and if the pain is relieved, a further 6 weeks non-weight-bearing with crutches is recommended. Of ten consecutive patients so treated, eight have remained free from pain after the resumption of full-weight-bearing. If microfractures are responsible, it is a reasonable hypothesis that these will unite during the 12 week period of freedom from stress.

Revision

Revision of a prosthetic hip is followed by a greater risk of complications than the primary operation. The surgery necessary to treat subsequent complications carries yet more risk (figure 13.38). Before embarking on the potentially hazardous venture of revision, the surgeon should consider the possibility of a Girdlestone arthroplasty, which may be the preferable alternative.

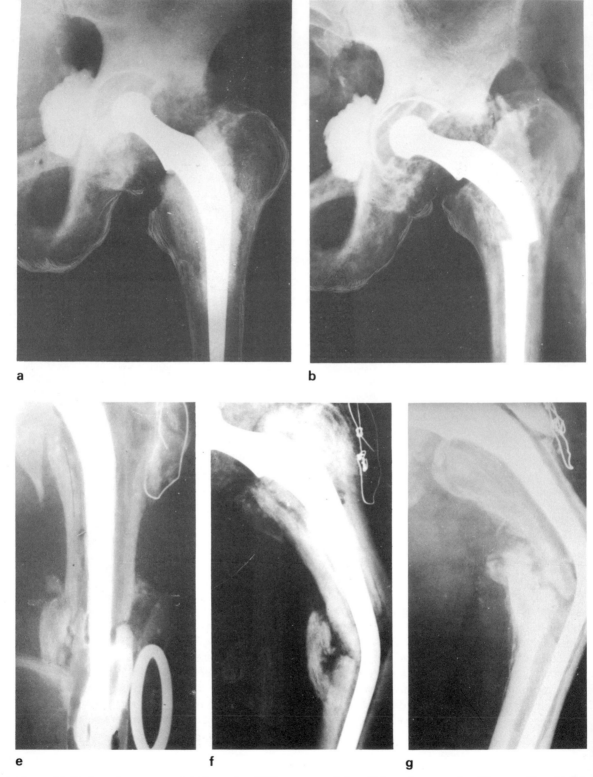

Figure 13.38 An unhappy saga: (a) November 1970—a successful total hip replacement in a 79-year-old male; (b) December 1974—sudden onset of pain with a fracture of the femoral stem; (c) February 1975—after revision for which the trochanter was removed. A long-stem prosthesis may have prevented further trouble; (d) November

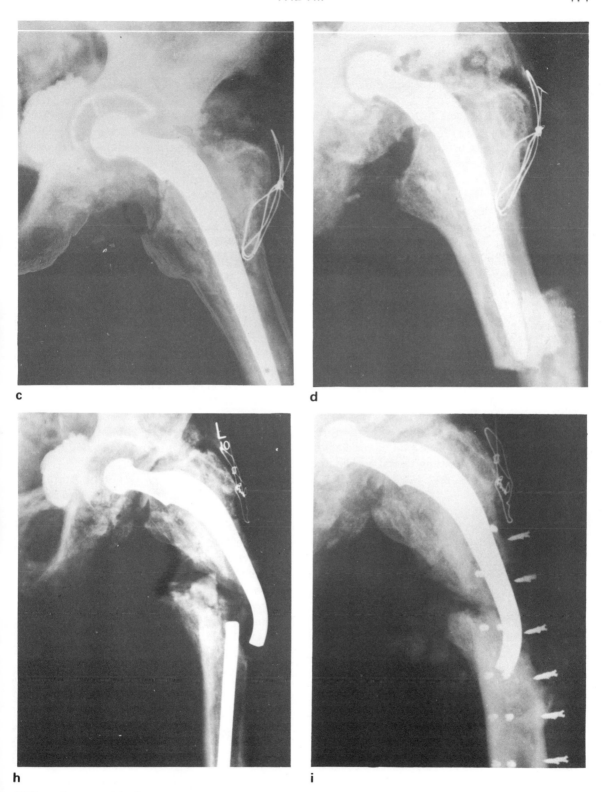

c
d
h
i

1975—a fracture of the femoral shaft at the level of the tip of the prosthesis; (e) December 1975—revision with a long-stem prosthesis. Traction was maintained for 3 months and then weight-bearing gradually commenced; (f) August 1976; (g) May 1977; (h) June 1978; (i) February 1979—Chichester instrumentation and iliac bone graft.

REFERENCES

Ansell, B. and Arden, G. P. (1979). *The Surgical Management of Juvenile Chronic Polyarthritis,* Academic Press, London

Bigvoet, O. L. M., Nollen, A. J. G., Slooff, T. J. J. H. and Feith, R. (1974). Effect of adiphosphanate on para-articular ossification after total hip replacement. *Acta Orth Scand.,* **45,** 926–934

Brooker, A. F., Bowerman, J. W., Robinson, R. A. and Riley, L. H. Jr (1973). Ectopic ossification following total hip replacement. *J. Bone Jt Surg.,* **55A,** 1629–1632

Boutin, P. (1972). Total hip arthroplasty made of dense ceramics. *Rev. Chir. Orthop. répar. Appar. moteur,* **58** (3), 229–246

Charnley, J. (1959). The lubrication of animal joints. *New Scientist,* July, 60

Eichler, J. (1973). A supporting ring to anchor the plastic cup for surgical treatment of protrusio acetabuli. *Med. Orth. Technik,* **93**(2), 28–31

Girdlestone, G. R. (1943). Acute pyogenic arthritis of the hip. Operation giving free access and effective drainage. *Lancet,* **i,** 419

Haboush, E. J. (1953). A new operation for arthroplasty of the hip based on biomechanics, photoelasticity, fast-setting dental acrylic and other considerations. *Bull. Hosp. Jt Dis.,* **14** (2), 242

Hardinge, K., Williams, W., Etienne, A., MacKenzie, D. and Charnley, J. (1977). Conversion of fused hips to low friction arthroplasty. *J. Bone Jt Surg.,* **59B** (4), 385–397

Haw, C. S. and Gray, D. H. (1976). Excision arthroplasty of the hip. *J. Bone Jt Surg.,* **58B,** 44–47

Jones, R. (1908). On the production of pseudarthrosis of the hip without disarticulation of the head. *Br. Med. J.,* No. 7, 1494

Lowe, L., Haran, F., Brozovic, M. and Fisher, M. (1976). An evaluation of small dose subcutaneous heparin in the control of deep venous thrombosis after hip arthroplasty. *6th Combined Meeting Orth. Ass. Eng. Speaking World,* London

McKee, G. K. and Watson Farrar, J. (1966). Replacement of arthritic hips by the McKee Farrar prostheses. *J. Bone Jt Surg.,* **48B**(2), 245

Milch, H. (1965). *Osteotomy at the Upper End of the Femur,* Williams and Wilkins, Baltimore

Osborne, G. V. and Fahrni, W. H. (1950). Oblique displacement osteotomy for osteoarthritis of the hip. *J. Bone Jt Surg.,* **32B,** 148

Partridge, A. (1976). Nylon straps for internal fixation of bone. *Lancet,* Dec 4, 1252

Partridge, A. (1977). Nylon plates and straps for internal fixation of osteoporotic bone. *Lancet,* April 9, 808

Pauwels, F. (1961). New principles for surgical treatment of coxarthrosis. *Verh. Dtsch. Orthop. Ges.,* 332

Read, J. (1967, 1978). Personal communication.

Rhys-Davis, H. and Benjamin, A. (1962). Unpublished research.

Ring, P. A. (1968). Complete replacement arthroplasty of the hip by the Ring prosthesis. *J. Bone Jt Surg.,* **50B,** 720

Russell, R. G. G. (1975). Diphosphonates and polyphosphonates in medicine. *Br. J. Hosp. Med.,* September, 297–314

Schatzker, J. and Hastings, D. (1976). Acetabular reinforcement in hip arthroplasty. *Rheum. Arth. Surg. Soc. Meeting,* Toronto

Smith-Petersen, M. N. (1935). Arthroplasty of the hip. A new method. *J. Bone Jt Surg.,* **21** (2), 269

Smith-Petersen, M. N. (1925). Joint ankylosis. Surgical methods for its prevention and relief. *Trans Interstate Postgrad. Med. Assembly of N. America.* St. Paul Minnesota, Oct.

Sweetnam, D. R., Mason, R. M. and Murray, R. O. (1960). Steroid arthropathy of the hip. *Br. Med. J.,* **1,** 1392

Wainwright, D. (1970). Upper femoral osteotomy. Robert Jones Lecture. *Br. Orth. Ass.,* Autumn Meeting.

Wiles, P. (1957–8). The surgery of osteoarthritis of the hip. *Br. J. Surg.,* **45,** 488

14

THE KNEE

The knee joint is capable of withstanding enormous loads, as may be readily appreciated by observing a downhill skier (figure 14.1). The correct alignment of the knee and its consequent stability depends on muscles, ligaments and body weight holding the normal contours of the tibial and femoral condyles in apposition. Damage to bone and soft tissue by rheumatoid disease will

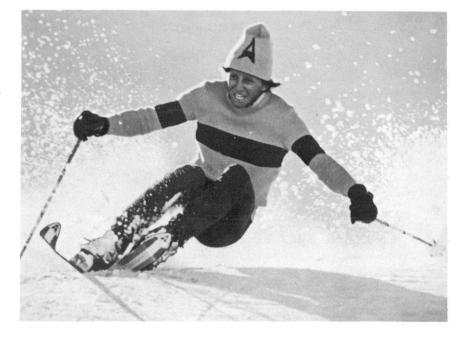

Figure 14.1 Stress and strain on the knees of a downhill skier (Farrell–Kästle)

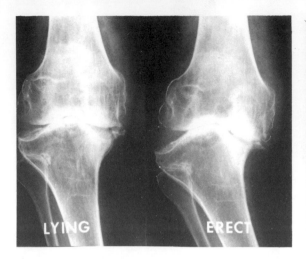

Figure 14.2 Weight-bearing X-rays reveal instability (G. Arden)

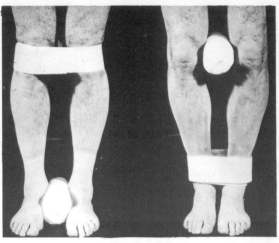

Figure 14.3 The Brattström stress method (H. Brattstrom)

upset this delicate balance, causing pain, instability and deformity. Proliferation of the synovium and damage to the capsule, ligaments, cartilage and bone are characteristic of rheumatoid disease in the knee; secondary osteoarthritic changes may supervene later. The onset may be insidious or rapid. It begins with a synovitis and is frequently bilateral. Pain is an early dominant feature, whereas loss of mobility occurs late in the disease. Instability due to damage of ligaments and bone leads to progressive valgus or varus deformity. Malalignment or flexion deformity is an indication for urgent treatment.

EXAMINATION

Synovial swelling, effusion, range of movement and instability are assessed, also vascularity in the lower limb, as there is a high incidence of rheumatoid vasculitis which may cause pain. X-ray examination must include anteroposterior weight-bearing or stress films of both knees (Brattström, 1976; figures 14.2 and 14.3). Long films indicate deviation of the mechanical axis when there is varus or valgus deformity (Waugh, 1977; figures 14.4 and 14.5). Flexion deformity is almost always present but not necessarily obvious, and may give

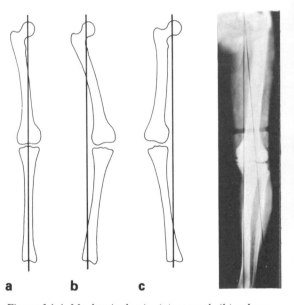

a   b   c

Figure 14.4 Mechanical axis, (a) normal; (b) valgus; (c) varus (W. Waugh)

Figure 14.5 Long X-ray film showing the mechanical axis drawn from the head of the femur to the ankle (W. Waugh)

misleading appearances of varus or valgus. The X-ray is affected by rotation at the hip joint. Internal rotation of the hips in the presence of knee flexion gives the appearance of valgus at the knee and external rotation gives the appearance of varus (figure 14.6).

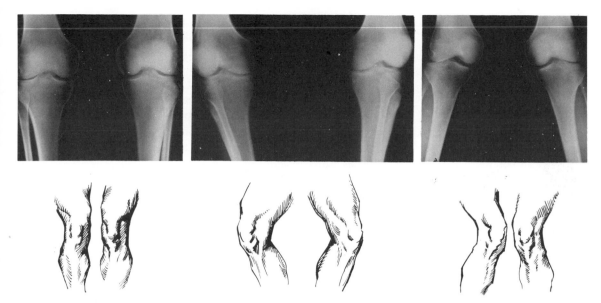

Figure 14.6 *The effect of hip rotation on the X-ray appearance of slightly flexed knees*

INSTABILITY

There are three types of instability of the knee:

(1) Medial or lateral ligament instability, in which the femoral and tibial condyles are undamaged and alignment of the knee is correct; this may be associated with occasional momentary giving way of the knee and is only diagnosed by collateral ligament stress tests when the patient is on the examination couch.

(2) Medial or lateral ligament instability with undamaged bony condyles combined with varus or valgus deformity due to skeletal malalignment; this results in an increase in deformity on weight-bearing and may be converted into type (1) by an appropriate osteotomy of either the tibia, the femur or both (figure 14.7).

(3) Instability may be due to destruction of the tibial or femoral condyles. When there is signifi-

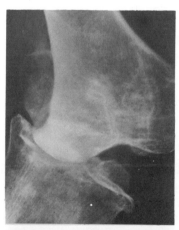

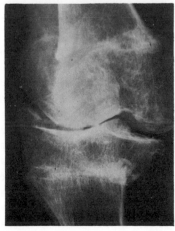

Figure 14.7 *(a) Medial ligament instability with valgus deformity and no condylar destruction; (b) weight-bearing X-ray after double osteotomy. Valgus has been corrected without removing wedges and functional stability is restored*

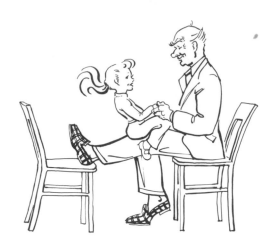

Figure 14.8 Passive correction of early flexion deformity

cant instability of this type, osteotomy is contra-indicated and prosthetic replacement is necessary (figure 14.2).

TREATMENT

Conservative treatment

Pain and increasing deformity are the important indications for treatment. The stresses due to muscular action and gravity increase with the degree of deformity and early recognition of increasing deformity is vital. When full extension is lost, the mechanical advantage of the quad-riceps muscle is diminished and that of the flexor muscles increased, resulting in progression of the flexion deformity. If the deformity is untreated, hamstring muscle action on the flexed knee results in posterior dislocation of the tibia on the femur and external rotation, owing to the turning moment exerted by the laterally placed biceps tendon insertion. The established classical triple deformity of the rheumatoid knee is one of flexion, posterior dislocation and external ro-tation of the tibia on the femur. This triad should never be allowed to develop; it is prevented by recognising the significance of minimal flexion

contracture and recommending simple con-servative treatment at that stage. The manage-ment of increasing early flexion deformity is perhaps the most important function of con-servative treatment. Active and passive extension exercises are necessary: active extension by powerful quadriceps contraction and passive ex-tension by weight applied over the knee with the heel supported on a chair (figure 14.8).

Quadriceps muscle exercise

An efficient quadriceps muscle protects the knee against the strains of everyday activity and will compensate for much of the instability due to ligament laxity, provided the bony structures are intact. Active quadriceps exercises may overcome slight knee flexion deformity and will prevent its development or recurrence. Quadriceps exercise, both in a physiotherapy department and at home, is the most important part of conservative treat-ment and is best practised isometrically with the knee straight; isotonic contraction aggravates patellofemoral arthritis. Quadriceps exercise is most effective in association either with heat, such as short-wave diathermy, or with ice packs applied over the knee joint; the most beneficial of these alternatives is found by trial. This treatment should be given in prescribed periods; chronic prolonged physiotherapy is of little value and should be avoided. Instruction in quadriceps exercises in the physiotherapy department enables them to be continued at home.

To encourage active contraction, a very short period of faradic stimulation is sometimes helpful, as also is maximal surge faradism, which improves poor quadriceps tone, increases its bulk and improves static contractability. This technique was developed from the treatment of stress incon-tinence by maximum perineal electrical stimu-lation (Moore and Schofield, 1976). Under general anaesthetic, and using a Rank selective treatment unit (Stanley Cox Ltd), a large stationary elec-trode is placed under the sacrum while a mobile disc stimulates the vastus medialis and rectus femoris each for 1 min. The faradic surge lasts 3 s with a similar rest period; the voltage is adjusted to produce maximum contraction. Following this, the electrodes are connected to a Bristow faradic

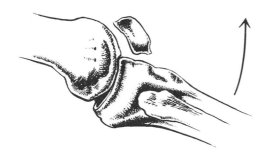

a

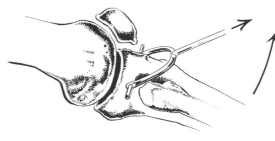

b

Figure 14.9 (a) Manipulative correction of severe flexion deformity damages cartilage and subchondral bone. (b) Traction forward on the tibial condyles while flexion is being corrected might prevent this

coil, with the core fully engaged and an unsurged faradic current given for 1 min to each of the two muscles. An immediate increase in thigh circumference of 12 mm ($\frac{1}{2}$ inch) was recorded in all but one of 14 patients treated consecutively. Routine isometric quadriceps contractions followed recovery from the anaesthetic and clinical improvement occurred in 13 cases (Gifford, 1977).

Plaster immobilisation

The acutely painful rheumatoid knee often responds to 4 week rest in a plaster cylinder with the knee fully extended. This may give prolonged relief of pain and make surgical intervention unnecessary. A plaster back-splint worn at night may help in treating a mild flexion deformity.

Flexion deformity

If the contracture is over 15°, osteotomy or prosthetic replacement is usually indicated. Manipulation under anaesthetic, or wedge plaster casts are not recommended, as the necessary pressure damages the subchondral bone. A method has been devised to correct the deformity by applying forward traction to the upper tibia while the knee is being extended, in an effort to avoid damaging the joint surfaces; although ingenious, it is generally ineffective (figure 14.9).

Steroid injection

The painful rheumatoid knee with synovial effusion may be aspirated and injected intra-articularly with local anaesthetic. Frequent injections of steroids are inadvisable, owing to the possibility of infection and Charcot-type joint damage (Sweetnam, Mason and Murray, 1960).

Operative treatment

There is no universal surgical panacea; the plethora of surgical procedures recommended is an indication not only of the many types and degrees of severity of knee disease, but also of the imperfections of these procedures.

The indications for surgical intervention are pain, loss of function and increasing deformity; the most important of these is pain. Constant rest-pain, day and night, is not only debilitating, but can also reduce the expectation of life.

Soft tissue release

Posterior capsulotomy and hamstring tenotomy for severe flexion deformity are unrewarding in adults, owing to the consequent loss of movement and the almost inevitable recurrence.

Ligament repair

The operative repair or reconstruction of ligaments in rheumatoid disease, either on its own or in association with prosthetic replacement, is usually of no value. The periarticular tissues are diseased and tissue transplanted from elsewhere, being anchored to diseased bone, in time becomes affected itself. Carbon fibre replacement of ligaments shows promise, but its value in rheumatoid disease has yet to be proven (Jenkins, 1978).

Patellectomy

The benefit gained from the removal of the patella seldom justifies the harm which results from its loss. Patellar impingement may complicate total knee replacement and should be treated by redesigning or re-inserting the prosthesis rather than removing the patella.

Débridement, cheilectomy and Pridie's procedure

Débridement and cheilectomy (Jones and Lovett, 1923), at one time favoured in the treatment of osteoarthritis and rheumatoid arthritis, are now almost forgotten. The removal of debris and irregular areas of cartilage and bone, as well as Pridie's procedure, which involves the removal of small circles of bare bone with a trephine to encourage fibrocartilage regeneration, may be beneficial (Pridie, 1959). There has been insufficient follow-up of these procedures for adequate assessment.

Synovectomy

Surgical synovectomy for the knee was first described by Volkmann in 1885; the vast literature on the subject and the conclusions as to the rightful place of synovectomy in the treatment of the rheumatoid knee are contradictory (chapter 4).

Indications

Anterior synovectomy is indicated in the presence of a persistent large effusion associated with thickened synovium which does not respond to conservative measures; another indication is a large popliteal cyst.

Contraindications

Bony damage, more than minor erosions, is considered a contra-indication by most surgeons, although some evidence supports the view that synovectomy is beneficial, even in the presence of

quite severe bone and cartilage damage (chapter 4).

Total or partial synovectomy

Partial anterior synovectomy is recommended, for the prevalent view in favour of total synovectomy is misconceived. Proliferative rheumatoid synovium has been compared to malignant tissue in that it appears to invade bone and erode it. This may be so, but, unlike malignant disease, any portion of synovium left after a sub-total synovectomy has no further tendency to invasion or spread. In fact, it appears to regress as thickened rheumatoid synovium does after osteotomy (chapter 5). Even if the entire suprapatellar pouch of diseased synovium is left *in situ*, it does not spread into the newly formed synovial joint cavity, which rapidly develops following partial synovectomy (Marmor 1976). We remove the suprapatellar pouch but do not mind leaving small areas of diseased synovium in less accessible places.

Popliteal synovial cysts

In rheumatoid disease these connect to the knee joint cavity through the posterior capsule, where the tissue planes form a valve allowing synovial fluid to pass from the joint into the cyst but not in the reverse direction. Radio-opaque dye injected into a suprapatellar pouch will appear in a popliteal cyst a few minutes after the patient has been allowed to walk, during which time (figure 14.10) the dye is pumped through the valve into the cyst. Surgical removal of a popliteal cyst is not advised, as it is technically difficult; the skin may heal with difficulty and the cyst may recur. A sub-total anterior synovectomy is almost invariably followed by total regression of the posteriorly situated cyst.

Rupture of a popliteal synovial cyst may be mistaken for a calf vein thrombosis. The clinical picture of the two conditions may be identical and they are differentiated by the history of acute onset in the case of the ruptured cyst (Dixon and Grant, 1964; Solomon and Berman, 1972).

Surgical technique

The knee joint is exposed through a straight midline anterior longitudinal skin incision; the capsule is incised medially, the incision extending

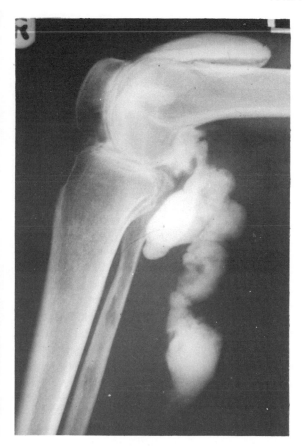

Figure 14.10 A popliteal cyst filled with dye after walking a few yards. The dye was injected into the suprapatellar pouch (G. Arden)

proximally into the rectus tendon rather than into the belly of the vastus medialis. As much of the diseased synovium as can easily be reached from this one incision is removed and the joint closed in layers. If suction drainage is used, the drain is removed within 24 hours. The limb is immobilised in a plaster cylinder with the knee straight for 3 weeks, after which mobilisation is commenced. If the knee does not regain mobility within 4 weeks from the operation, it is manipulated under a general anaesthetic.

Results

Synovectomy may be followed by many years of freedom from pain. It appears that the results of synovectomy become progressively less satisfac-

tory as the degree of bone and cartilage damage increases, although some authorities contest this view (chapter 4).

The prepatellar bursa

When the prepatellar bursa has to be excised, every care is necessary to avoid sepsis, as the bursa may sometimes connect with the joint cavity. Immobilisation of the knee in a plaster of Paris cylinder for 10 days after the operation aids skin-healing.

Osteotomy

Osteotomy relieves pain, serious complications are rare, and, if unsuccessful, it may be followed by prosthetic replacement. The correction of deformity during prosthetic replacement may be difficult or even impossible, and in such cases, so long as there is union in improved position the osteotomy previously performed facilitates the subsequent total replacement. A remarkable result of double osteotomy is that swollen, hot rheumatoid synovium shrinks dramatically and clinically returns to normal (Benjamin, 1969) within 6 weeks of operation. Osteotomy adjacent to the knee may be through the tibia, the femur or both. It may relieve pain both in the deformed knee and in the knee without deformity. There is evidence in our practice to indicate that a rheumatoid knee with a small degree of varus can do well with a tibial osteotomy on its own, whereas the valgus knee and the knee with neither deformity is better treated by double osteotomy.

Double osteotomy

The main indication for double osteotomy is severe pain which has failed to respond to conservative treatment. The presence or absence of deformity does not alter this indication. When there is no deformity, non-displacement osteotomies are undertaken, and when there is deformity, it is fully corrected. In view of the correction taking place at two sites, double osteotomy is particularly suitable for more severe degrees of valgus (figure 14.11), varus deformity and any flexion deformity; Volkmann in 1874 made this observation in correcting gross deformity after tuberculosis of the knee. When the

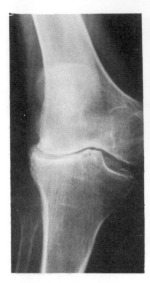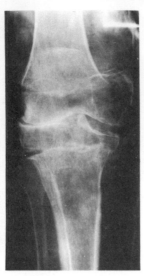

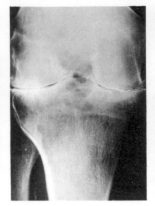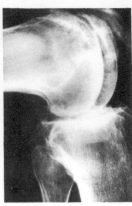

Figure 14.12 A very narrow joint-space, but a good range of movement and so a suitable case for osteotomy

Figure 14.11 Valgus corrected by double osteotomy. The correction taking place at both osteotomy sites. No wedges

arthritic changes are principally in the patello-femoral compartment, pain is relieved by double osteotomy and patellectomy is seldom recommended.

Contra-indications

Instability due to bone destruction is the main contra-indication. The rheumatoid knee is unable to maintain stability, even with good alignment, when one of the femoral or tibial condyles is destroyed. Following double osteotomy the range of movement is almost invariably reduced by a few degrees, and consequently a preoperative range of under 45° is generally a contra-indication and 90° is desirable. An expectation of life of less than 5 years contra-indicates this procedure, owing to the long post-operative recovery time compared with the rapid return of function following a total prosthetic replacement. Loss of joint-space as seen on X-ray, however severe, is not a contra-indication if there is 90° range of movement (figure 14.12). Areas of bone denuded of cartilage, seen at operation, are consistent with a satisfactory result (figure 14.13).

Operative technique (figure 14.14)

With the patient supine, the limb exsanguinated and the surgeon standing on the opposite side, a straight midline longitudinal anterior skin incision is made from below the tibial tuberosity to above the upper border of the patella (figure 14.14e). The incision is deepened through the capsule, medial to the patella, down to bone, without reflecting flaps. The patella and patellar tendon are dislocated laterally and the tibial condyles exposed subperiostially, separating from bone the upper 25 mm (1 inch) of the origin of the anterior tibial group of muscles. The knee is flexed fully and remains so, whenever the knife or osteotome is in use, to ensure that the popliteal artery drops away from the posterior joint capsule and so is less vulnerable to damage (figure 14.14a and b). The tibia is osteotomised above the insertion of the patellar tendon, 25 mm (1 inch) distal to the articular margin of the tibia. With the knee flexed, bone levers are passed on either side of the tibial condyles, a narrow osteotome cuts through the lateral cortex and then a broad osteotome is driven across from the medial cortex to meet the narrow osteotome already in position. The posterior tibial cortex has probably not been divided, and the osteotomy is completed by hinging the tibial condyles on the posterior cortex and so breaking it. This hinging is achieved by using two osteotomes as levers. If deformity is to be cor-

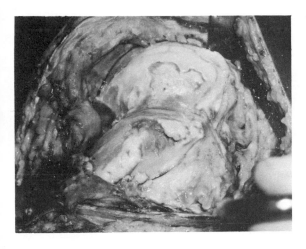

Figure 14.13 Denuded areas of femoral cartilage but suitable for osteotomy

rected, the knee is extended and manipulated into the desired position; one side of the osteotomy crushes and the other opens up. The consistency of the bone in rheumatoid disease allows this correction to take place and the removal of a wedge is never necessary. The patella is redislocated and with the knee flexed bone levers are inserted on either side of the lower end of the femur. The femoral osteotomy site is at the widest part of the femoral condyles, and is thus not merely within the knee joint but distal to the most proximal portion of the articular cartilage. Care is taken that the osteotomy is at a right angle to the femoral shaft such that it remains entirely in the cancellous condylar bone and does not extend to the shaft posteriorly. The osteotomy is undertaken in a similar fashion to that of the tibia. Any residual deformity that is uncorrected at the tibial osteotomy is corrected at the femoral by manipulation, again with the knee straight. It is advisable to overcorrect deformity by a few degrees, as the joint always opens a little and apparent correction is due partly to ligamentous laxity. The tourniquet is released and the capsule approximated with a few interrupted sutures to hold the patellar mechanism in place. Care is taken when suturing the skin to protect its blood supply, particularly at a point just below the patella. Here there is a danger of some skin necrosis, which may

be avoided by using Allgover Basle or subcuticular sutures. A well-padded plaster cylinder is applied from the groin to above the ankle and as this sets the centre of the ankle, the centre of the knee and the head of the femur are aligned (figure 14.4a), taking care to avoid undue skin pressure. An X-ray is taken immediately. If the desired position has not been achieved, the plaster cast is wedged while the patient remains anaesthetised.

Post-operative care

Full weight-bearing is allowed immediately, but crutches are permitted for a few days should the patient need them. Between the fifth and sixth week the patient is re-admitted to hospital, the plaster is removed, full weight-bearing permitted and knee flexion immediately encouraged. If a range of flexion of 30° has not been achieved within 2 days, the knee is gently manipulated under anaesthesia. The threat of manipulation motivates the patient actively to flex the knee. Ninety degrees is almost invariably achieved within a few weeks. Physiotherapy aggravates the arthritis at this stage in treatment, and we do not recommend it unless a flexion deformity is developing.

Complications

Serious complications are rare. We have seen two tibial (figure 14.15a) and no femoral non-unions in 600 personal double osteotomy operations. A case of femoral non-union which has been shown to us had been osteotomised proximally in the suprapatellar pouch and a wedge had been taken (figure 14.15b and c). An area of skin necrosis sometimes occurs adjacent to the wound, just below the patella (figure 14.16), which may expose bone but always heals spontaneously. The innocuous nature of skin necrosis overlying an osteotomy is in striking contrast to the serious problem of such necrosis over a prosthetic joint replacement. Following osteotomy, lack of correction of valgus or varus deformity, although undesirable, is consistent with pain relief. Sometimes, however, residual varus deformity results in medial joint-line pain which can be relieved by further corrective tibial osteotomy.

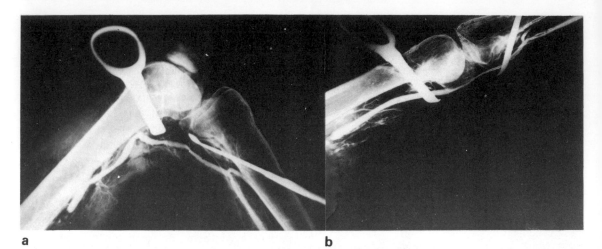

a   b

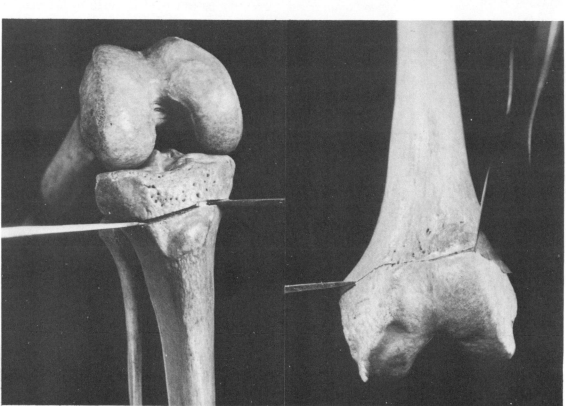

c   d

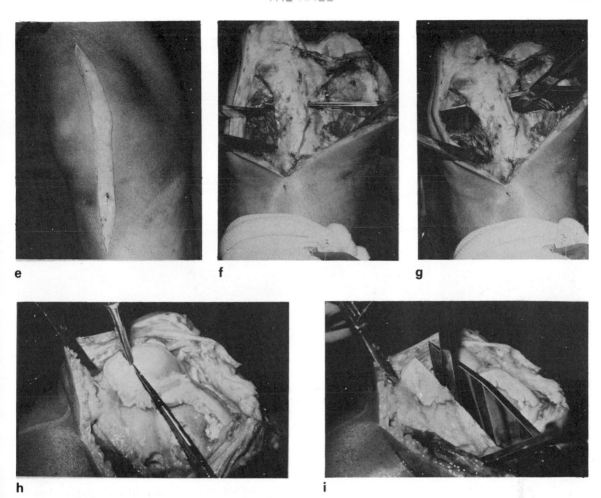

Figure 14.14 Double osteotomy technique: (a) Arteriogram of recent cadaver lower limb—the flexed knee allows the popliteal artery to drop away from the posterior joint capsule; (b) the artery is adjacent to the capsule when the knee is extended and it is in danger of being trapped by bone levers and of being cut by an osteotome; (c) the tibial cut above the quadriceps insertion; (d) the femoral cut crosses articular cartilage; (e) midline incision; (f) the tibial cut—the two osteotomes meet; (g) the posterior cortex is broken by opening the osteotomy with the two osteotomes; (h) the femoral cut; (i) completion of the femoral osteotomy

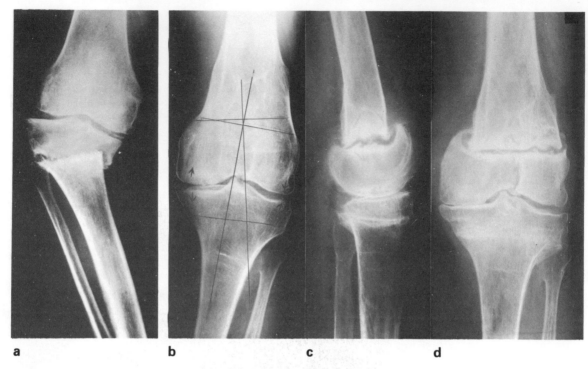

a   b   c   d

Figure 14.15 (a) Non-union of a tibial osteotomy; (b) a wedge measured to correct varus. It is unnecessary and too far proximal; (c) and (d) non-union of the femoral osteotomy

Results

Pain is relieved for over 5 years in 79 per cent of cases (figure 14.17). Objectively the range of movement is never increased following operation, although the patient thinks so when pain is relieved. Following a successful double osteotomy, the X-ray appearance gradually improves although no increase in joint space is seen, disuse atrophy reverses and the internal bony structure as seen on X-ray improves. A review at 9–16 years after operation of 50 patients who had been pain-free at 5 years, revealed that 36 remained free from symptoms and 14 had recurrence of pain, at times varying from 6 to 15 years. Several series of double osteotomy operations performed in different centres have now been assessed and they have an overall good result of approximately 70 per cent. A careful breakdown of the results is now necessary to enable better preoperative selection of patients (table 14.1). Significant factors may be age, erythrocyte sedimentation rate, sero-positive or sero-negative, long-term steroid therapy and psychological state, as well as varus or valgus deformity and range of movement (Benjamin, 1976). Our evidence suggests that the most favourable results are achieved in patients under 50 years of age, sero-negative, with an ESR of under 40 and with minimal or no deformity (Benjamin and Crabtree, 1977); nevertheless double osteotomy is frequently indicated in the absence of these favourable criteria.

Rationale

It is suggested that the success of osteotomy, in relieving arthritic pain, may result not only from alteration of the lines of forces which pass through a joint, but also from biological change resulting from section of bone and soft tissues. This is postulated in view of the relief from pain expressed by patients immediately following intertrochanteric osteotomy before weight-bearing, and following double osteotomy even in the absence of deformity or if existing deformity is not corrected. 'Even more curious is the dramatic shrinkage of rheumatoid synovium in the early weeks following

TABLE 14.1 DOUBLE OSTEOTOMY OF THE KNEE 1961–73, ASSESSED IN 1976 (A.B.)

206 knees in 177 patients:	osteoarthritis 127 (42 ♂, 85 ♀) rheumatoid arthritis 79 (10 ♂, 69 ♀) Valgus 48; Varus 80; Neither 78
Indications:	Severe knee pain owing to OA or RA unrelieved by prolonged conservative treatment.
Contra-indications:	Instability owing to bone deficiency; combined medial and lateral instability; insufficient range of movement; less than 1 year life expectancy.
Good result:	Slight or no pain and no more than 15° loss of pre-operative range of movement.

RESULTS

Good 154 (76%)   Not good 52 (24%)

		Osteoarthritis		Rheumatoid arthritis	
		Good	Not good	Good	Not good
Male	Valgus	7	0	0	0
	Varus	21	6	5	1
	Neither	8	0	4	0
Female	Valgus	20	5	13	3
	Varus	26	11	7	3
	Neither	17	6	26	17

		Valgus		Varus		Neither	
		Good	Not good	Good	Not good	Good	Not good
Male	OA	7	0	21	6	8	0
	RA	0	0	5	1	4	0
Female	OA	20	5	26	11	17	6
	RA	13	3	7	3	26	17

	Good		Not good	
Age	OA	RA	OA	RA
30–39	1	2		
40–49	12	8	2	3
50–59	26	10	7	9
60–69	41	29	15	9
70–79	13	6	4	3
80–89	6			

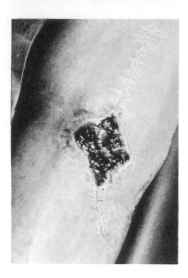

Figure 14.16 An area of skin necrosis adjacent to the patellar tendon. This is prevented by a midline incision, incising straight down to the bone and joint and careful skin suturing

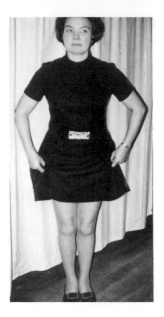

Figure 14.17 Photograph taken in 1976 of a patient who had a double osteotomy of one knee in 1961 and the other in 1962. She had been disabled, unable to walk for 2 years by knee pain due to strongly sero-positive rheumatoid arthritis

operation. We suggest that the intraosseous pressure of articular bone in arthritis is raised, with sinusoidal pooling (figure 14.18) and that osteotomy reduces the pooling thus lowering the raised pressure (Brooks and Helal, 1961; Arnoldi, Lemperg and Linderholm, 1971; Helal, 1962).

Single osteotomy

In certain cases it may be sufficient to correct deformity by either a tibial or a femoral osteotomy. A knee with slight varus and little or no flexion deformity responds to a tibial osteotomy, whereas the valgus knee does not (Harding, 1976; Coventry, 1975). A dome or Brackett osteotomy (figure 14.19) (Brackett, 1912) is advised, and if adequate correction cannot be attained, then either the fibula is osteotomised or its head is excised. There are theoretical reasons why femoral osteotomy on its own might be suitable in certain cases but there is insufficient clinical evidence to support this. It is not known whether a single osteotomy would benefit a rheumatoid knee without deformity. A horizontal knee joint when the patient is erect may be a factor in achieving a painless knee, although, once again, there is insufficient evidence to support this attractive theory (chapter 5). If this is important, it indicates

whether a corrective osteotomy is better done at the tibia, at the femur, or both.

Bone and cartilage transplant

The transplantation of total knee joints from the cadaver has not proved a practical procedure. Laurence (1976) has reported six cases; the donors were under 40 years of age and the tissues had been typed. Failure was due to tissue rejection. Imamaliev (1969) emphasises the importance of overcoming tissue incompatability and of correct storage conditions.

Forty osteochondral allografts from recent cadavers have been reported by Gross (Gross *et al.*, 1976). The tissues are typed, there is no immunosuppression and no rejection has occurred (figure 14.20). Osteochondral allografts may prove of value in the rheumatoid knee, although so far they have been used in osteoarthritis only.

Prosthetic replacement

The objectives in knee replacement are pain relief,

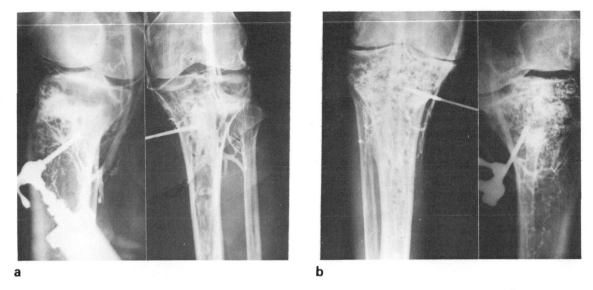

Figure 14.18 Tibial venograms. (a) a normal knee; (b) an arthritic knee—the deep veins are larger, sinusoids are closely packed, they appear more rotund and extend into the subchondral area. The dye is forced further down the medulla

Figure 14.19 Dome or Bracket osteotomy: (a) drill-holes mark the intended line of osteotomy; (b) and (c) the osteotomy is complete and varus has been corrected. The fibula osteotomised at a lower level

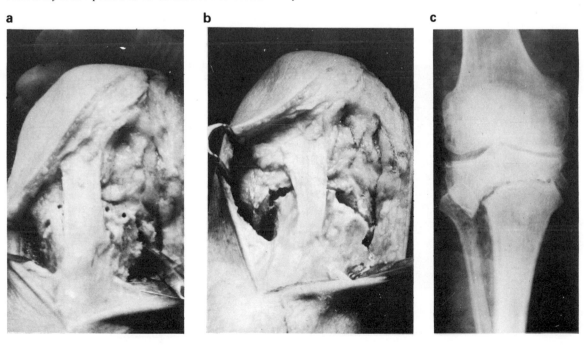

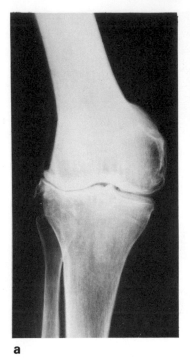 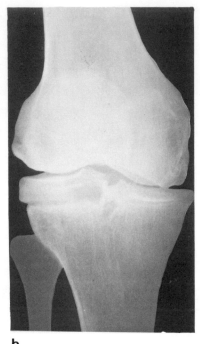 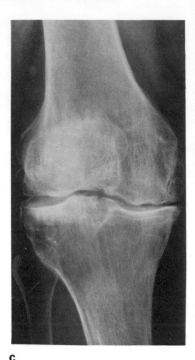

a   b   c

Figure 14.20 Osteochondral allograft (A. Gross): (a) before operation; (b) 1 month later; (c) 2 years after operation. The graft is incorporated and standing films are straight

Figure 14.21 The Platt prosthesis

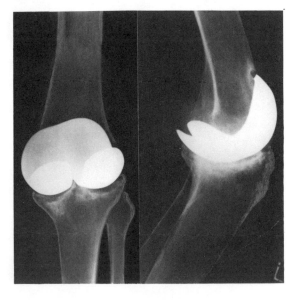

restoration or preservation of motion, correction of deformity and restoration or preservation of stability.

Partial prosthetic replacement

Partial prosthetic replacement may be femoral, tibial or patellar. The Platt femoral prosthesis is a stainless steel metal shell which fits over the femoral articular surface (figure 14.21). It is no longer in use and is of historic interest only. Patellar prostheses, which provide a covering for the articular surface of the patella, are still experimental and not in general use.

There are successful tibial joint surface replacements, although we do not make general use of them in our practice. The MacIntosh plateau prosthesis provides a useful means of dealing with the painful rheumatoid knee, without the more serious complications of the total prostheses and does not preclude subsequent total prosthetic replacement. Whereas in degenerative arthritis a unicompartmental operation is satisfactory, in rheumatoid disease both tibial articular surfaces must be replaced by prostheses. MacIntosh (1967) considers that correct posterior placement of the prosthesis gives

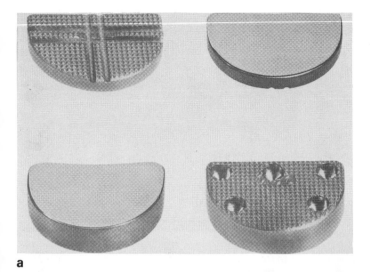

a

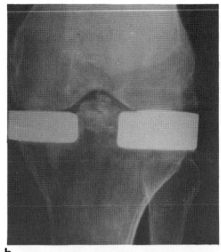

b

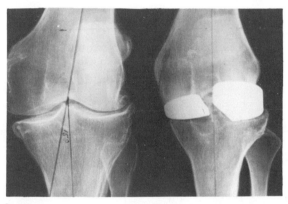

c

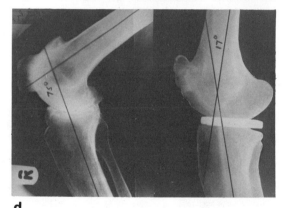

d

*Figure 14.22 MacIntosh plateau (A. Kates): (a, b)
Kates modification of the MacIntosh plateau—
obtainable from The London Splint Co.; (c) correction
of valgus deformity by using prostheses of different
thicknesses; (d) correction of flexion deformity by using
a thin prosthesis and removing a little more subchondral
bone*

adequate fixation but, in view of the loosening
which may occur, Kates (1973) has modified the
MacIntosh prosthesis by a series of roughened
drill-holes on the undersurface so that it can be
cemented in place (figure 14.22a, b). In the
severely damaged rheumatoid knee, extensive
destruction of the femoral condyle may leave virtually no intercondylar notch. A new intercondylar notch should be gouged out; otherwise
weight-bearing will be on the tibial spine and not

on the prosthesis. It is possible to correct minor
degrees of valgus or varus deformity by inserting
prostheses of various thicknesses (figure 14.22c).
Flexion deformity may be decreased by the insertion of a thin plateau after excising the tibial joint
surfaces (figure 14.22d).

Total replacement

There are over 200 designs of total prosthetic knee
available to the surgeon. None of these is as
satisfactory as a successful hip prosthesis and none
is designed to withstand vigorous activity. Knee
prostheses may be constrained, unconstrained or
partially constrained. These terms are not precise
but indicate the torsional stress which is likely to
fall upon the cement–bone interface.

The hinge knee prostheses permit flexion and
extension only, without rotation, and are called

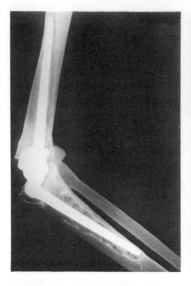
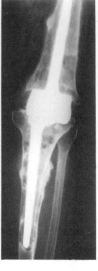

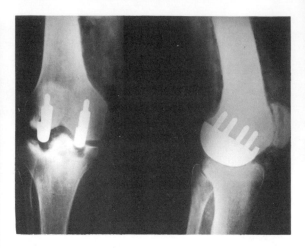

Figure 14.24 The Gunston polycentric knee prosthesis (G. Arden)

Figure 14.23 Loosening of a Shiers hinge prosthesis. There are stress fractures and cystic changes. This knee was revised and there was no infection (G. Arden)

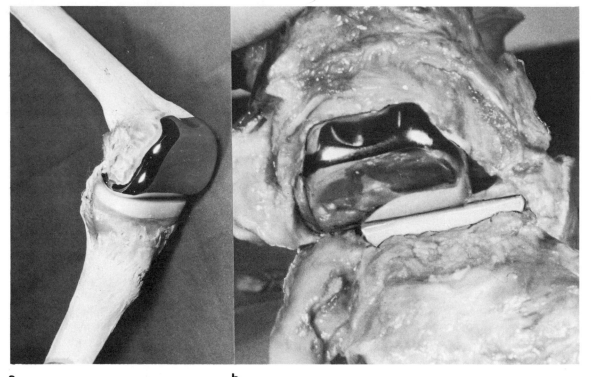

a   **b**

Figure 14.25 The Freeman–Swanson prosthesis: (a) almost unconstrained and relies on intact ligaments and accurate alignment for stability (M. Freeman); (b) a cadaver specimen. The prosthesis was inserted 4 years previously. Malalignment is the cause of the femur sliding off the tibia

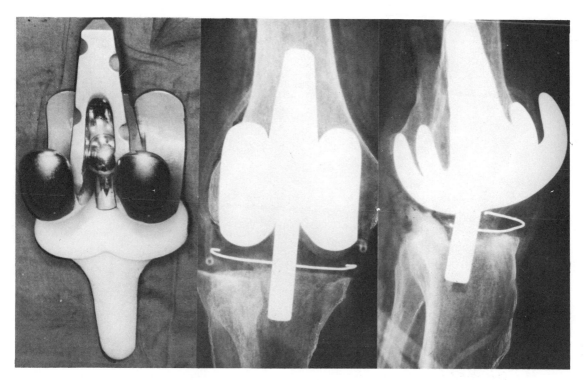

Figure 14.26 The Attenborough knee (G. Arden)

'constrained'. As rotational stresses are taken at the cement–bone interface they are liable to loosen (figure 14.23), although the results of the Stanmore hinge appear encouraging (Lettin *et al*., 1978).

The large group of total prostheses in which the femoral and tibial components are not linked vary in their degree of constraint. The greater the curvature of the articular surfaces the greater the constraint, as the femoral runners tend to be held within the groove in the tibial component by body weight and muscle tension (figure 14.24). The comparatively flat Freeman–Swanson prosthesis is almost entirely unconstrained (figure 14.25a). We have used this prosthesis, and, in our hands, have sometimes found it difficult to insert with the joint surfaces perfectly horizontal. If the unconstrained prosthesis is inserted with the joint surface sloping, a gradual subluxation of the femoral component on the tibial occurs (figure 14.25b).

A third series is now being developed which is partially constrained; the Attenborough (figure 14.26) and Sheehan (figure 14.27) prostheses are examples and we have experience of the latter (Sheehan, 1974). This prosthesis allows rotation when the knee is flexed and gradually becomes more constrained as the knee is extended. We find the Sheehan knee obeys many of the criteria for a satisfactory prosthesis. Not too much bone has to be removed for its insertion, so that an arthrodesis can be undertaken should the prosthesis have to be removed. The prosthesis is buried deep in the intercondylar femoral notch, thus being less likely to endanger the nutrition of the overlying skin. Patellar impingement does not appear to be a problem, although patellar realignment may be necessary in the valgus knee. Its range of over 95° of flexion permits the rheumatoid patient with poor upper limbs to stand up from the sitting position without too much difficulty (figure 14.28). The cemented intramedullary stems are a disadvantage but are for stability. Our Sheehan replacement knees reviewed at 4–5 years reveal some failures due to central tibial stub breakage and others in which the polyethylene wear has been excessive. Lack of correction at operation of either valgus or varus predisposes to these failures.

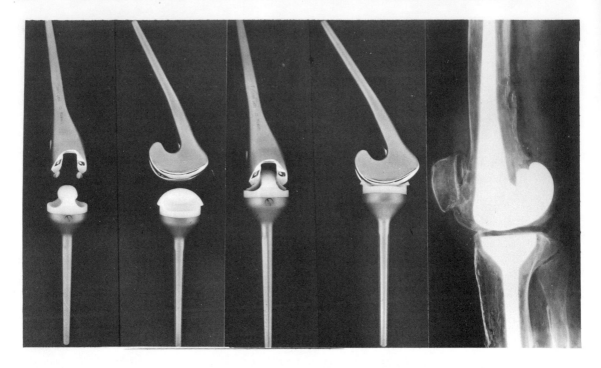

Figure 14.27 The Sheehan knee (J. Sheehan)

Considerable biomechanical skill and ingenuity is devoted to the design of the many prosthetic knees now being developed. As well as the constrained hinges, there are condylar replacements or coverings, modified hinges, uniaxial and polyaxial joints of various designs

Figure 14.28 Bilateral Sheehan knee replacement. Flexion beyond 90° enables the rheumatoid patient to stand up with the assistance of the upper limbs

and retropatellar coverings. The names given to these designs can be confusing. The terms 'Geometric' and 'Geomedic' are apparently synonymous and eponyms cause confusion when the same name is retained for a series of different designs of knee from the same source.

Indications for prosthetic knee replacement

Pain associated with a degree of instability and bone destruction uncontrolled by a lesser procedure is the main indication for prosthetic replacement.

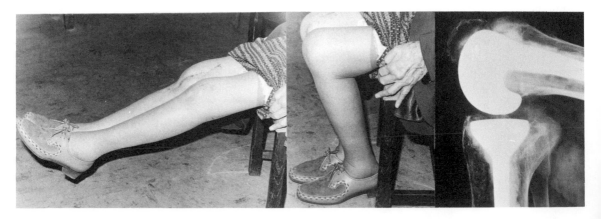

The Sheehan prosthesis operative technique

Our exposure differs somewhat from Sheehan's. Instead of a medial parapatellar incision we make a longitudinal straight midline skin incision (figure 14.14e). The capsule is incised medially, and the patella is displaced and rotated so that the articular surface points laterally as the knee is flexed. Without this rotation the skin margin may remain in the wound as a possible cause of septic contamination. If the patellar ligament starts to tear from bone during this displacement, tension may be relieved by extending the incision superiorly into the quadriceps muscle or rectus tendon. The knee remains fully flexed during the operation. The femoral intercondylar notch is widened and the shaft reamed to accept the femoral component, which sits deeply into the notch. A circular disc of bone and cartilage is removed from the articular surface of the tibia, and the shaft and condyles are reamed to accept the tibial component. Both components have stems and are cemented after trial insertion. As the femoral component is inserted, it links with the tibial, which is already in place. The specially designed jigs are essential, but experience is still necessary for the correct placing of the prosthesis (figure 14.29).

After the cement is set and the knee put through its range of movements, the head of the table is tilted downwards and the tourniquet released. Sheehan suggests an interval of between 8 and 10 min between the setting of the cement and release of the tourniquet. He also suggests an intravenous injection of 50 mEq. of bicarbonate, prior to the tourniquet release, to counteract acidosis. We do not follow the latter suggestion, but consider it important to maintain adequate circulating blood volume. These measures prevent the occasional hypotensive collapse, which follows release of the tourniquet, possibly due to toxic effects of free monomer from the cement (Risung, 1976). Suction drainage is recommended; the skin is closed with interrupted Allgover Basle or subcuticular sutures and a pressure bandage is applied.

Technical points applicable to many prostheses

The designer's detailed instructions should be studied and kept available in the operating theatre. The less experienced surgeon will find that the femoral medullary cavity is more posterior than expected and the tibial more anterior. The medial tibial cortex is more vulnerable to damage than the lateral and it is advisable to displace the tibia slightly medially when drilling it.

Normally the foot is rotated 20° externally, in relation to the knee, but it is usually advisable, when inserting a total prosthesis into a valgus knee to rotate the tibia internally a little in relation to the femur. Post-operative valgus deformity frequently occurs when this advice is ignored. External rotation of the tibia on the femur exaggerates valgus and internal rotation exaggerates varus. Correction of the rotation may be all that is necessary. To correct valgus or varus deformity, extensive soft tissue release may be necessary and is achieved by sub-periosteal dissection of the femoral attachments of the medial or lateral collateral ligament. There is little latitude to vary the position of prostheses with intramedullary stems and correction should be complete, before the insertion of the prosthesis, so that force is not needed in maintaining the correction while the cement is setting. Severe valgus, varus or rotation deformities may be corrected by preliminary osteotomy, several months before total replacement.

Considerable surgical skill is necessary to achieve the accurate alignment required when inserting a partially constrained or unconstrained knee prosthesis.

Patellar malalignment should be corrected by the appropriate release and reefing of the quadriceps expansions. The patellar tendon insertion occasionally requires transposition.

Fixed flexion deformity is usually corrected by sinking the tibial component more deeply. Posterior soft tissue release is not advised, and if sufficient bone is resected to correct fully a fixed flexion, then the stability of the knee is endangered. A residual deformity of 20° usually corrects spontaneously in the few weeks after operation. Full extension of the other knee is necessary to ensure this spontaneous correction, and in the event of bilateral fixed flexion of more than 20° both knees should be operated upon with an interval of 2–3 weeks, for otherwise the oper-

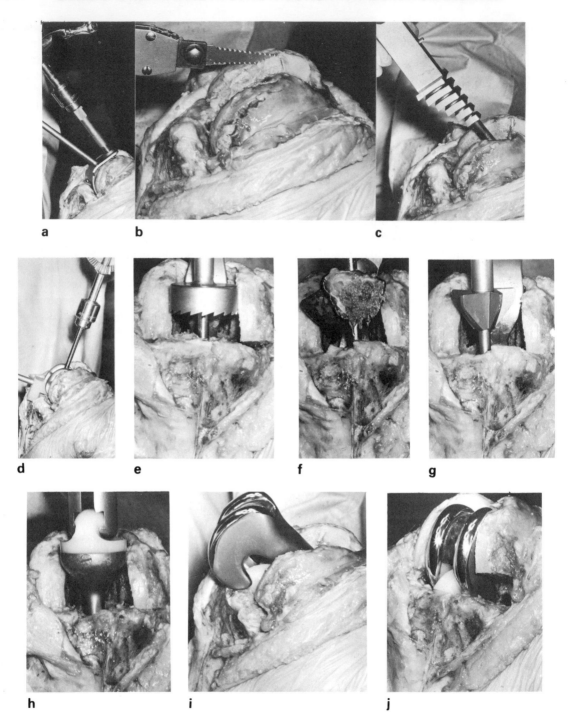

Figure 14.29 Sheehan knee operative technique: (a) femoral jig and drilling of femoral medulla; (b) widening of intercondylar notch; (c) the femoral reamer; (d) the tibial jig and drilling of tibial medulla; (e) the tibial disc reamer passing through widened femoral intercondylar notch; (f) removal of block of tibial bone; (g) the tibial reamer; (h) the insertion of the tibial component; (i) the insertion of the femoral component; (j) the two components engaged

ated knee would assume the position of the unoperated knee.

Post-operative management

The foot is rested on plastic foam to reduce flexion deformity. The suction drain is removed at 24 hours, when static quadriceps exercises are commenced, and the outer dressings removed on the fourth day, when flexion is started. On the seventh day the wound is inspected and partial weight-bearing with crutches is allowed.

Contra-indications to total replacement of the knee

(1) Peripheral vascular disease, including vasculitis.

(2) Neuropathy.

(3) Disorder of the quadriceps mechanism. Knee arthroplasty is dependent on the quadriceps muscle, and a patient with any derangement of the extensor mechanism, including a previous patellectomy, should be approached with caution, whereas a non-functioning quadriceps is an absolute contra-indication.

(4) Previous arthrodesis. We do not advise the conversion of a sound painless arthrodesed knee to an arthroplasty.

(5) Previous infection.

(6) Persistent foci of chronic infection, such as indolent varicose ulceration and desquamating psoriasis, increase the probability of early and late deep infection.

(7) Poor skin overlying the anterior aspect of the knee may break down, with consequent failure of the prosthesis. This is more likely in the presence of long-term steroid therapy.

(8) Uncorrected angular deformity of the bones.

(9) Uncorrected fixed hip deformity (figure 13.17, p. 157).

(10) If bone destruction is severe, the partially constrained prostheses may not be satisfactory, and one of the hinge prostheses with intrinsic stability may have to be considered; however, we feel the constrained hinge should not be used if it can be avoided.

(11) Any condition of the knee which is likely to respond to synovectomy or osteotomy.

(12) Still's disease. A special femoral component is necessary which uses the same bearing surfaces but all of the other dimensions are reduced.

Complications

(1) Inadequate correction of fixed deformity, in particular valgus. Several degrees of fixed deformity are consistent with several years of painless activity, but any malalignment must throw unnecessary strain on the prosthesis and the cement—bone interface. Every effort should be made at operation to avoid it.

(2) Skin breakdown rarely occurs, but in the severe rheumatoid with atrophic skin from long-term corticosteroids, great care is necessary, as wound breakdown may mean sacrifice of the prosthesis (figure 14.30). Secondary healing may occur without this sacrifice, by treating such cases in a back-splint, avoiding active knee flexion until the wound has healed.

(3) Cracking of femoral condyle. The major problem is loss of alignment, and provided this is prevented, the cement will act as an internal splint and an uninterrupted recovery is likely to take place, although full weight-bearing should be delayed by a few weeks.

(4) Deep infection. If this occurs, the prosthesis and the cement must be removed by anterior guttering. Sufficient cancellous bone should remain to allow for a compression arthrodesis. Prostheses that do not allow for this should not be

Figure 14.30 Skin necrosis (a) and consequent exposure; (b) of a total knee prosthesis after 4 years of painless activity (G. Arden)

a   b

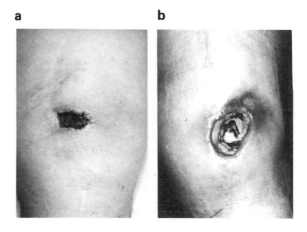

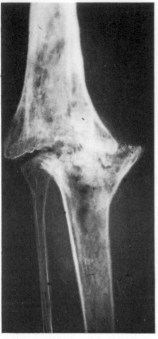
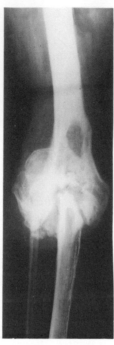
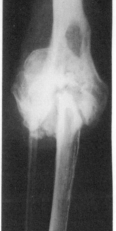

a

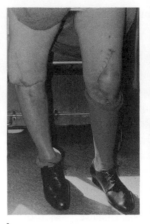
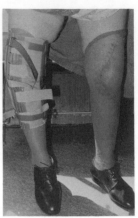

b

Figure 14.31 (a) Non-union after an attempted arthrodesis following failure of a total knee replacement; (b) a brace sometimes enables the patient to walk a few steps

used. Rarely, deep infection can be eliminated by systemic antibiotic in association with prolonged local irrigation of the antibiotic.

(5) Patellar problems. Several of the prostheses in current use need redesigning, owing to patellar impingement. Patellofemoral problems are unusual following the Sheehan replacement. Patellectomy should always be avoided.

(6) Loosening. The incidence of late complications, particularly loosening, increases every year and body weight appears to be a significant factor. Loosening of the prosthesis occurs earlier in heavier patients.

Arthrodesis

Primary arthrodesis of the knee, seldom indicated in rheumatoid disease, is technically simple but the Charnley compression method (Charnley and Lowe, 1958) requires care, to prevent damage to porotic bone, whereas staple fixation is effective and avoids the external device (chapter 7). Arthrodesis of the knee as a salvage procedure following the failure of a total prosthetic replacement is difficult to achieve (figure 14.31a). As more knees are replaced by prostheses, the problem of

salvage for painful loosening and infection will increase. In the event of deep infection, attempts to save the prosthesis usually fail and early removal is advisable. To remove the cement, guttering of both tibia and femur is necessary and an X-ray required to confirm complete removal of barium-containing cement. Debris and fibrous tissue are removed from between the bone-ends, which are nibbled back to expose bleeding cancellous tissue. The two surfaces are compressed with clamps applied to skeletal transfixing pins. Two tubes are inserted, one for suction and the other for instilling an antibiotic or bactericidal agent. These tubes may be kept *in situ* for several weeks. Fibrous union is often all that can be achieved, but is sufficient to allow walking with an external brace; in time, bony union may occur (figure 14.31b).

CONCLUSION

Help may be provided for the painful rheumatoid knee by a wide variety of surgical procedures. Selection of the most suitable procedure for each patient is vital but the correct choice of operation requires considerable knowledge, experience and judgement. It is unfortunate that emphasis is placed at present on prosthetic design and that biomechanical symposia consider the prosthesis first and the patient's problems second, or not at all.

Fifty per cent of all walking difficulties in rheumatoid disease are attributable to the knee joint. Over 90 per cent of such patients will be relieved by medical treatment and simple physiotherapy such as local heat and exercise. Most of the resistant knees will respond to synovectomy or osteotomy, operations rarely associated with complications. Moreover synovectomy or osteotomy, for the majority of patients, offers many years of freedom from pain; additionally, a knee so treated is able to withstand the stresses and strains of normal activity, including running and jumping. A total knee prosthesis will permit an elderly patient sedentary activity but will be quite unsuitable for the stresses of normal active life. Total prosthetic replacements should be reserved for the small group of patients who are resistant to less radical measures. Our views on the choice of treatment are indicated in table 14.2 depicting a hypothetical series of painful arthritic knees.

No surgeon can be fully conversant with the multitude of procedures described for rheumatoid disease of the knee, and therefore the operation selected depends partly upon the condition of the knee and partly upon the preference and experience of the surgeon. In our departments, four procedures are commonly used; table 14.3 summarises our indications for each procedure.

TABLE 14.2 HYPOTHETICAL SERIES

	Knee pain due to arthritis 500 CASES		
Treatment	Pain relieved	Not relieved	Serious complications
Conservative	400(80%)	100(20%)	0
Osteotomy in 100 cases not relieved by conservative treatment	70(70%)	30(30%)	1
Prosthesis in 30 cases not relieved by osteotomy	26(86%)	4(14%)	2(0.4%)
Final results Original 500	496(99.2%)	4(18%)	1
Immediate prosthesis	430(86%)	70(14%)	25(5%)

TABLE 14.3 SURGICAL INDICATIONS FOR THE RHEUMATOID KNEE

Clinical features	Radiological features	Operative procedure
Persistent synovial proliferation and effusion	Minimal bony changes	Synovectomy
Pain and varus deformity	Changes mainly medial compartment	Tibial or double osteotomy
Pain with valgus or no deformity	Changes mainly lateral or in all compartments, including patello-femoral	Double osteotomy
Pain with valgus, varus or flexion deformity of over 30°		Double osteotomy
Pain after osteotomy or other conservative procedure		Total prosthesis
Pain with less than 45° range of flexion		Total prosthesis
Pain with severe instability	Destruction of one condyle, femoral or tibial	Total prosthesis
Pain with a life expectancy of less than 5 years		Total prosthesis

REFERENCES

Arnoldi, C.C., Lemperg, R. K. and Linderholm, H. (1971). Immediate effect of osteotomy on the intramedullary pressure of the femoral head and neck in patients with degenerative arthritis. *Acta Orth. Scand.*, **42**, 454–455

Benjamin, A. (1969). Double osteotomy for the painful knee in rheumatoid arthritis and osteoarthritis. *J. Bone Jt Surg.*, **51B**, 694

Benjamin, A. (1976). Tape slide presentation. *Combined meeting Br. Am. Orth. Assoc.*, London

Benjamin, A. and Crabtree, S. (1977). Assessment of double osteotomy of the knee. In preparation.

Brackett, E. G. (1912). A study of the different approaches to the joint with special reference to the operation for curved trochanteric osteotomy and for arthrodesis. *Boston Med. J.*, **166**, 235

Brattström, H. (1976). Personal communication.

Brooks, M. and Helal, B. (1968). Primary osteoarthritis, venous engorgement and osteogenesis. *J. Bone Jt Surg.*, **50B**, 493–504

Charnley, J. and Lowe, H. G. (1958). A study of end results of compression arthrodesis of the knee. *J. Bone Jt Surg.*, **40B**, 633

Coventry, M. B. (1975). Osteotomy of the upper portion of the tibia for degenerative arthritis of the knee. *J. Bone Jt Surg.*, **47A**, 984

Dixon, A. St J. and Grant, C. (1964). Acute synovial rupture in rheumatoid arthritis. *Lancet*, 742–745

Gifford, D. (1977). Physiotherapist Enfield District Hospital. Personal communication.

Gross, A. E., Langer, F., Haupt, J., Pritzher, K. and Friedlander, G. (1976). Allotransplantation of partial joints in the treatment of osteoarthritis of the knee. *Clin. Orth.*, **108**, 7–14

Harding, M. L. (1976). A fresh appraisal of tibial osteotomy for osteo-arthritis of the knee. *Clin. Orth. Related Res.*, **114**, 223–234

Helal, B. (1962). Osteo-arthritis of the knee joint. M. Ch. Orth. Thesis

Imamaliev, A. S. (1969). The preparation, preservation and transplantation of articular ends. *Recent Advances in Orthopaedics*, Churchill, London, pp. 209–263

Jenkins, D. H. R. (1978). The induction of new anterior cruciate ligaments in sheep and the clinical use of filamentous carbon fibres in the human. *Br. Orth. Ass. Combined Meeting*, September

Jones, Sir R. and Lovett, R. W. (1923). *Orthopaedic Surgery*, Frowde, Hodder and Stoughton, London, p. 262

Kates, A. (1973). Personal communication

Laurence, M. (1976). Transplantation of articular cartilage *Rheum. Arth. Surg. Soc. Meeting*, Toronto

Lettin, A. W. F., Deliss, L. J., Blackburne, J. S. and Scales, J. T. (1978). The Stanmore hinged knee arthroplasty, *J. Bone Jt Surg*, **60B**(3), 327–332

MacIntosh, D. L. (1967). Arthroplasty of the knee in rheumatoid arthritis using the hemiarthroplasty prosthesis. *Synovectomy and Arthroplasty in Rheumatoid Arthritis* Second Int. Symp. (Ed. G. Chapchal) Stuttgart. Thieme.

Marmor, L. (1976). *Arthritis Surgery*, Lea and Febiger, Philadelphia, p. 341

Moore, T. and Schofield, P. F. (1976). The treatment of stress incontinence by maximum perineal electrical stimulation. *Br. Med. J.*, **3**, 150–151

Pridie, K. H. (1959). A method of resurfacing osteoarthritic knee joints. *J. Bone Jt Surg.*, **41B**, 618

Risung, F. (1976) Toxicity of cement. *Mtg Rheum. Arth. Surg. Soc. Meeting*, Boston

Sheehan, J. (1974). Personal communication

Solomon, L. and Berman, L. (1972). Synovial rupture of the knee joint. J. *Bone Jt Surg.*, **54B**, 460–467

Sweetnam, D. R., Mason, R. M. and Murray, R. O. (1960). Steroid arthropathy of the hip. *Br. Med. J.*, **1**, 1392

Volkmann, R. Von (1885). Chirurgische erfahrungen über die Tuberculose. *Verhandlungen der Deutschen Gesellschaft für Chirurgie*, Vol. 14, Ch. VII.

Volkmann, R. Von (1874). Osteotomy for knee joint deformity. *Berlin Klin. Wehnsche.*, No. 50, 629–631

Waugh, W. (1977). Personal communication

15

THE ANKLE AND FOOT

The ankle and foot are prime sources of difficulty in walking. This perhaps is not fully appreciated, judged by the vast literature devoted to problems of the hip and knee as compared with those of the foot. An assessment conducted at the London Hospital on a consecutive series of rheumatoid patients who had walking difficulties, demonstrated the following distribution of joints primarily responsible: hip, 2 per cent; knee, 53 per cent; ankle and hind-foot 20 per cent; fore-foot 25 per cent. Thus the ankle and foot together account for almost half the walking problems of the rheumatoid patient.

SYNOVITIS

On all aspects of the ankle joint are synovial tissues which can be involved in rheumatoid arthritis.

The Achilles tendon

The Achilles tendon itself may become involved in rheumatoid inflammation. Peritendinitis is best treated by rest in an equinus position, which will allow the inflammation to settle; simply raising the heel of the shoe may be helpful. Occasionally, rupture of the tendon occurs and can be treated surgically, or conservatively by an equinus plaster, non-weight-bearing for 4 weeks, followed by a weight-bearing plaster for 4 weeks with the ankle at right angles. Decision upon which course to adopt can be made as follows: if there is a gap palpable with the ankle in equinus, an operation is preferred; if the gap closes, operation is unnecessary.

There are two bursae, one superficial and the other deep to the insertion of the Achilles tendon. If symptoms arise from these, local injections of steroid can be tried, combined with a heel raise to take tension off the heel cord. If recurrent bouts of bursitis occur, or there is a persistent bursal tumour, then excision is justified.

Peroneal tenosynovitis

Swelling and tenderness is situated in the line of these tendons, behind the external malleolus, running forwards and downwards to the lateral side of the foot. Eversion against resistance will precipitate pain. Local injections of steroid may be helpful, but if swelling and pain persist, surgical decompression of the peroneal tunnel and synovectomy are carried out. The peroneal tendons may be impinged upon and compressed by the fibular malleolus in the presence of hind-foot valgus deformity. This may give rise to troublesome symptoms, and decompression can only be fully accomplished by resection of the apex of the fibular malleolus and decompression of the peroneal tunnel. A small synovial joint between the peroneal sesamoid and the calcaneum can be involved in rheumatoid synovitis. We have on two occasions had to excise this sesamoid and clear the joint of synovium to relieve symptoms.

The extensor compartment

Synovial involvement of the extensor tendons anterior to the ankle can be troublesome and entrapment under the retinaculum may occur. This may result in extrinsic tendon imbalance and account for some toe deformities. Decompression and synovectomy are sometimes indicated.

The tarsal tunnel

This lies behind the internal malleolus and descends to enter the plantar aspect of the foot. It contains the toe flexors, the tibialis posterior tendon and the posterior tibial nerve; synovitis here may be troublesome. If it does not respond to rest and steroids, then decompression and synovectomy may be necessary. Occasionally the posterior tibial nerve is entrapped and compressed by the synovitis, giving rise to pain and paraesthesiae in the sole of the foot, for which decompression is mandatory. The occasional small synovial joint between the posterior tibial tendon sesamoid and the navicular bone can be involved in rheumatoid disease. Excision of the sesamoid and synovial clearance is indicated when the pain, which is usually well localised, is persistent.

Bursae

The constant bursa situated between the tendon of the tibialis posterior and the plantar calcaneonavicular or spring ligament can be involved in rheumatoid synovitis, and if resistant to conservative measures, its removal offers a satisfactory relief of symptoms. Pain under the heel-pad may arise either from the bursa described or from a plantar fasciitis.

Large bursae arising from the synovial joints in the foot produce erosive destruction of the surrounding bone; these are not unlike popliteal cysts, in that they are usually valved, with fluid passing out of the joint into the bursae but not in the reverse direction. They are best dealt with by synovectomy or joint excision.

Synovitis of the ankle joint

This joint is infrequently involved early in rheumatoid disease. Joint swelling is best seen from behind, when the normal hollows on either side of the Achilles tendon disappear. Failure to respond to local steroid injection is an indication for a period of rest in a below-knee plaster cast. Longer-term rest is achieved by a below-knee double iron with square heel socket and a sole rocker bar to compensate for the loss of ankle movement. Patients willing to use such a device gain dramatic relief of pain, often after a few weeks rest in a brace of this type. Synovitis can be treated by limited synovectomy with an occasional rewarding result especially if tarsal fusion is being performed. If there is much destruction of the ankle joint, then a fusion will often provide a satisfactory outcome with certain provisos (see below).

THE ANKLE AND HIND-FOOT

These must be considered together, as their joints (namely the ankle, subtalar and midtarsal) are closely linked. The synovial linings of these and their surrounding tendons and bursae may be involved in rheumatoid disease, causing difficulty in pin-pointing the correct site of symptoms. Hind-foot deformity, particularly valgus, may be created in a number of ways and has to be carefully assessed for corrective treatment to be effective. The ankle, subtalar and midtarsal joints may be involved either individually or together in rheumatoid disease. These three joints are subject to stresses similar to those on the major proximal joints in the lower limb.

Hind-foot symptoms and signs

Pain arising from the ankle joint is poorly localised to the front of the ankle and to both sides. Swelling of the ankle is best observed from behind but may be visible anterior to the malleoli.

Subtalar joint pain is often referred laterally in front of the external malleolus.

Talonavicular pain is generally well localised and is either on the medial or the dorsal aspect of this joint. The talonavicular joint is often involved early and may be the first of these three joints to exhibit symptoms and signs.

Symptoms behind the ankle may arise in the Achilles tendon or its deep or superficial bursae. Stretching the tendon or compressing the adjacent structures by dorsiflexion of the foot aggravates these symptoms and placing the foot in equinus eases them. There is also local tenderness and the bursae involved may be palpable.

Symptoms on the medial side may arise in the tarsal tunnel, resulting from synovitis of the tibialis posterior and toe flexor tendon sheaths. Ankle pain may also arise on the medial side.

Rarely, entrapment of the posterior tibial nerve, in the tarsal tunnel, gives rise to paraesthesiae or numbness felt in the sole of the foot. Associated with medial compartment tenosynovitis, there may rarely be spasm of the muscles causing flexion of the toes and inversion of the foot, but such spasm is more commonly due to hysteria. Resisted inversion and flexion of the foot and toes generally aggravates symptoms if these are originating from the medial compartment.

Anterior pain may arise in the ankle joint and sometimes from tenosynovitis of the extensor compartment tendons.

Pain arising laterally

In an analysis of pain in the rheumatoid hind-foot, carried out at the London Hospital by Freeman and King (1975), it was shown that pain commonly arises on the lateral side of the hind-foot (figure 15.1). There are three sources for this pain: tenosynovitis in the peroneal compartment, impingement of the fibular malleolus against the os calcis and disease in the subtalar joint. In all three conditions the hind-foot tends to a valgus attitude. There may be spasm of the peroneal muscles, and passive foot inversion often gives rise to pain; resisted eversion of the foot, producing pain,

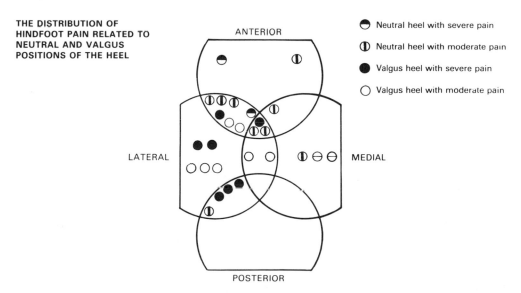

Figure 15.1 Distribution of pain in the hind-foot. There is clearly a lateral side preponderance

suggests a peroneal tenosynovitis. When subtalar pain is felt laterally, it is generally anterior and inferior to the external malleolus. Pain and tenderness beneath the heel, usually anterior or anteromedial on the heel-pad, arises from plantar fasciitis, which can be an early presenting symptom of rheumatoid arthritis.

In assessing the range of passive movement at the various joints in the hind-foot, it is important to anchor the adjacent joints. In assessing ankle movement, it is important to place the thumb on the neck of the talus, to be sure movement is taking place between the talus and the ankle mortise. In assessing subtalar movement, the ankle malleoli are held and the heel is rocked medially and laterally. In the normal foot there is little lateral movement, for most of the movement is medial. When testing the midtarsal joint, the heel should be anchored firmly and passive inversion/eversion and dorsiflexion/flexion movements attempted at the midtarsal joint.

Pain under the heel

Plantar fasciitis may be a presenting symptom of rheumatoid arthritis, gout or ankylosing spondylitis. The conservative treatment of fasciitis includes a valgus support, intrinsic foot exercises, faradic foot baths, local steroid injection, ultrasonic therapy and systemic anti-inflammatory drugs such as naproxen. Persistent pain, despite these measures, is an indication for a Steindler type of fasciotomy; this can be performed with a tenotome. Rarely, deep X-ray therapy has been prescribed with benefit for resistant cases.

The valgus hind-foot (figure 15.2)

This is the common deformity in the rheumatoid foot and its analysis is important for treatment to be effective (figure 15.4).

Valgus collapse may occur in the ankle joint itself (figure 15.3a), there may be subluxation at the talonavicular joint, the head of the talus moving medially and allowing the fore-foot to collapse into valgus (figure 15.3b). These may lead to fibular bending and fracture. Finally, the deformity may occur at the subtalar joint (figure 15.4c).

TABLE 15.1 CAUSES OF PAIN ABOUT THE ANKLE AND HINDFOOT

Site	Pathology
Posterior	Tendo-achilles tenosynovitis, bursae
Medial	Tarsal tunnel tenosynovitis, posterior tibial nerve compression, ankle and talo-navicular joint pathology
Anterior	Extensor tendon tenosynovitis, ankle and talo-navicular joint pathology
Lateral	Peroneal tendon tenosynovitis, lateral malleolus impingement, ankle and subtalar joint pathology
Heel	Plantar fasciitis, plantar bursae

In the normal foot there is a riding-up of the posterior subtalar facet on the adjacent facet of the calcaneum occurring as the subtalar joint is moved into inversion. In eversion the talus again descends and comes to a stop as the anterior facet of the talus approaches the corresponding facet on the calcaneum (figure 15.5). In rheumatoid disease, the bones are seen to contact and erosion of this 'buffer' occurs. Subtalar valgus, however,

Figure 15.2 Valgus hind-foot. It is not possible to be certain at which joint this is occurring without careful analysis

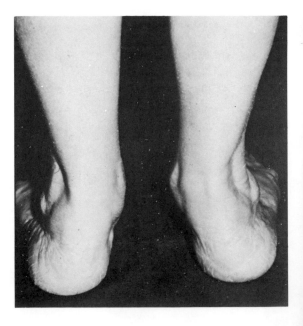

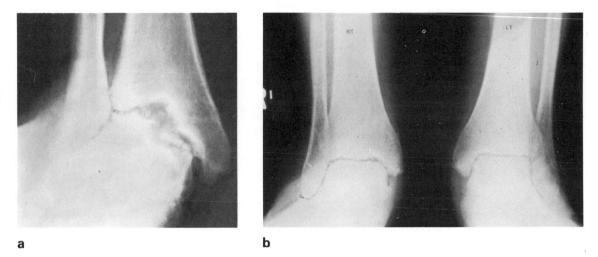

a   b

Figure 15.3 (a) X-ray—the valgus is clearly due to collapse of the ankle joint; (b) X-ray—the valgus is not occurring at the ankle but below. In fact the deformity is at the midtarsal joint

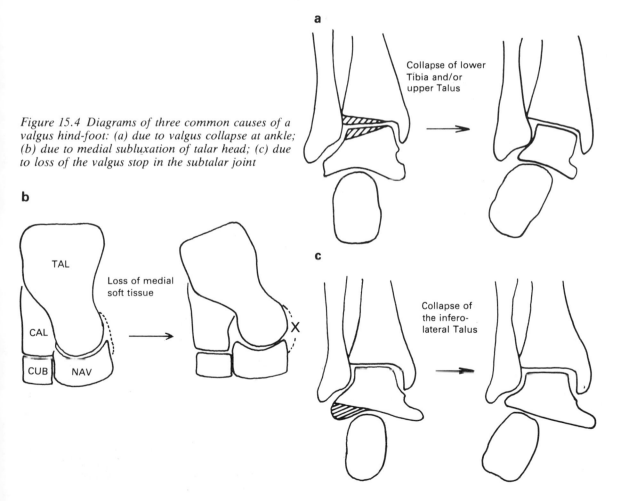

Figure 15.4 Diagrams of three common causes of a valgus hind-foot: (a) due to valgus collapse at ankle; (b) due to medial subluxation of talar head; (c) due to loss of the valgus stop in the subtalar joint

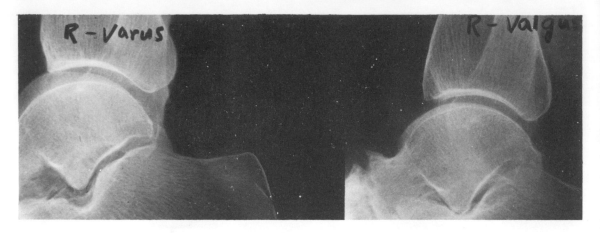

Figure 15.5 Inversion (varus) and eversion (valgus) views show how the anterior facet of the talus ascends and descends on to the calcaneum

probably starts as a result of disturbed sensory receptors, and consequent loss of tone in muscles such as the tibialis posterior, normally a dynamic factor preventing heel valgus (Samuelson, 1977).

Fibular impingement upon the calcaneum (figure 15.6)

This may occur due to valgus deformity. The pain will be aggravated by eversion of the foot. Subtalar disease causes pain not only on eversion of the foot, but also on inversion. In fibular impingement, the pain is felt at the site of impingement; that is, at the tip of the lateral malleolus. A further aid to diagnosis is a peroneal tenogram, which may show hypaque held up at the site of fibular impingement (figure 15.7). If treated by excision of the tip of the malleolus, temporary relief of pain is followed by further drift into valgus.

Realignment of the mobile valgus hind-foot

The deformity can be helped in the early stages by splintage. If the valgus is at ankle level, then a below-knee iron with a square socket in the heel and an inside T strap, or a double iron with square sockets and T straps is advised to prevent ankle movement and hold the foot in inversion; ankle movement is compensated for, by placing a rocker on the sole of the shoe (figure 15.8). Valgus at subtalar level can be treated by a similar device with a round socket on the shoe heel, to allow

ankle movement. Alternatively, a moulded plastic support extending from the knee to the forefoot is sometimes sufficient to control pain and deformity (figure 15.9); although not as rigid as a caliper, it is cosmetically superior.

Surgical management of the valgus hind-foot

Valgus at the ankle joint due to talar collapse on the lateral side, can be treated by arthrodesis of

Figure 15.6 This weight-bearing X-ray shows contact between the fibula and the calcaneum

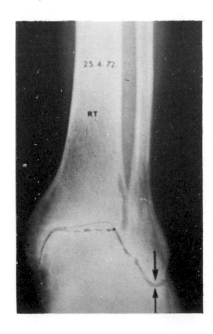

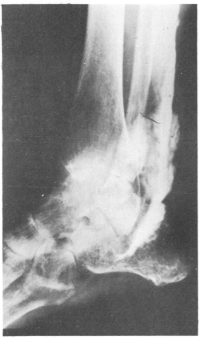

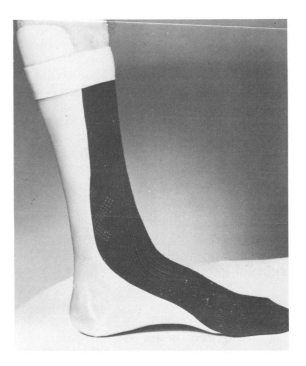

Figure 15.7 The peroneal tenogram shows compression of the soft tissues where there is calcaneofibular contact. This is part of the cause of pain

Figure 15.9 A moulded plastic support from below knee to metatarsal heads will control the mobile mild valgus deformity

Figure 15.8 Iron and T strap and rocker on shoe to compensate for loss of ankle movement

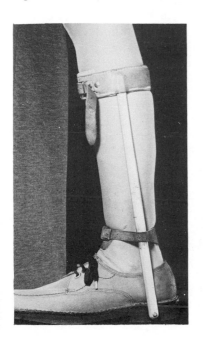

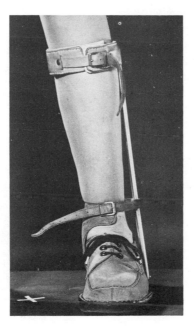

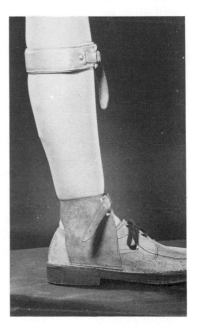

the joint in correct alignment. Alternatively, the joint can be replaced; this may eventually prove to be the procedure of choice. Valgus occurring at the subtalar joint can be treated by a fusion in the corrected position; full correction in severe deformity is difficult to achieve. An alternative surgical treatment is insertion of a so-called valgus-stop prosthesis, which prevents valgus and still allows subtalar movement. At the midtarsal joint, there is a choice between arthrodesis and replacement of the talonavicular joint.

Surgical management of the ankle and subtalar joint

Arthrodesis

The management of the ankle in polyarthritis differs considerably from that of monarticular disease, such as the degenerative ankle joint disease subsequent upon old injury or septic arthritis, when other lower limb joints are likely to be healthy and mobile. In the latter situation arthrodesis is the treatment of choice. It should be noted that in rheumatoid disease, spontaneous intertarsal fusions are relatively common, but natural ankle fusions are rare, and when they occur spontaneously, tend to be confined to chair- or bedridden patients. Ankle arthrodesis, even in the presence of a mobile tarsus, carries the risk of throwing additional stress on joints which may become involved by disease later (Kirkup, 1974; 1977). If both ankles are arthrodesed and the tarsus is stiff, then getting out of a chair is difficult, great stress falls upon the knees and any knee arthritis will be aggravated. It will be seen, therefore, that the prime indication for the development of a satisfactory replacement ankle joint is in rheumatoid arthritis.

Arthrodesis of the subtalar and midtarsal joint complex is principally indicated for pain and skin pressure problems and rarely for deformity alone. Arthrodesis to correct valgus may result in the foot relapsing into valgus at the ankle or distally; it is best reserved for the neutral foot with an intact ankle joint.

Prosthetic replacement

No-one, as yet, has much experience of ankle joint replacement, for few have inserted more than a score of these prostheses.

The first ankle joint implant was carried out by Buchholz in Hamburg some 8 years ago (Buchholz, Engelbrecht and Siegel, 1973). He had the first joint of his own design implanted into his own arthritic ankle: perhaps the ultimate gesture of good faith in a prosthesis.

The prostheses (figure 15.11) fall into two groups, dependent on their restriction of collateral shift—that is, in the provision of malleolar bearing surfaces or not. One of us (B. H.) designed and tested a total ankle joint in 1968. The tests indicated that collateral support is essential (figure 15.10) (see also Kempson, Freeman and Tuke, 1975). The TPR total ankle (P. D. Thompson) provides no significant malleolar buttress. The Smith and the St Georg (Buchholz) are domed. The ICLH (Freeman, Tuke and Samuelson, 1975) and the Mayo (R. N. Stauffer) provide built-in malleolar articulating surfaces. Experience at the London Hospital is confined to the ICLH (Imperial College London Hospital) prosthesis (figure 15.11). Our impression is that generally, pain relief is satisfactory. Movement on the whole is limited to a $20°-40°$ arc. All these prostheses can be salvaged by arthrodesis. A third type of joint designed by Lord and Marotte (1973) in France replaces ankle and subtalar surfaces of the talus. The prosthesis consists of a metal ball on a stem which is cemented into the tibia and a polythene

Figure 15.10 1968 experimental ankle prosthesis. The convex section should be metallic and vice versa

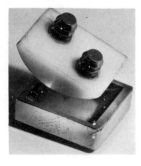

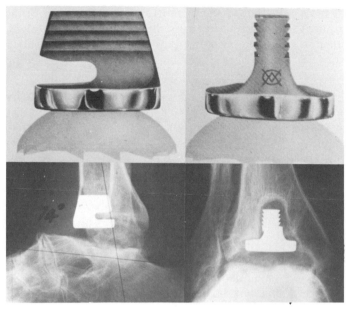

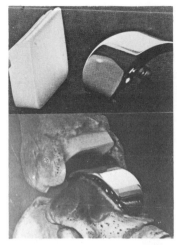

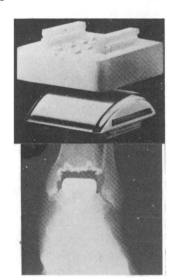

a

Figure 15.11 (a) Smith domed ankle. No collateral support. (b) TPR Thompson ankle. No collateral support. (c) St George. (d) Mayo. Collateral support. (e) ICLH. Collateral support

b

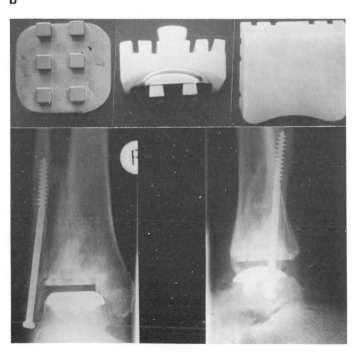

c

d

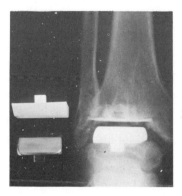

e

cup cemented into the calcaneum. Twelve cases are reported. One-third 'of the patients required subsequent correction of heel varus by tendon transposition and only three of the twelve were assessed as having good results at 2 years.

The subtalar valgus stop (Freeman et al., 1977)

The device consists of a polythene talar component and a metal calcaneal component. Both have flat surfaces and small stems, which are inserted into the respective bony surface. Valgus deformity is corrected and subtalar movement preserved (figure 15.12). A. Viladot of Barcelona, Spain, has used a silastic spacer in the tarsal tunnel for the correction of childrens' valgus feet and P. Grassin of Rennes, France, has used a stemmed metal stop inserted into the talus in the sinus tarsi of children.

Talonavicular joint replacement (Freeman and Tuke, 1975)

The talonavicular joint is sometimes involved in isolation early in rheumatoid disease. Valgus may occur because of medial subluxation of the head of the talus. A joint replacement will correct this and relieve pain (figure 15.13).

Combined talonavicular replacement and valgus-stop procedure

Frequently the valgus hind-foot, due to loss of valgus stop, may be combined with talonavicular arthritis, and the two problems can be dealt with by the insertion of the valgus-stop implant together with a talonavicular implant (figure 15.14).

Complications of ankle and hind-foot prosthetic joints

Faulty technique and inexperience may cause malpositioning and malalignment of the implant, necessitating revision of the procedure, while loosening necessitates re-cementing. Infection in one ankle was salvaged by removal of the prosthesis and arthrodesis.

Ankle and hind-foot osteotomies

Aside from the arthroplasties mentioned above, a number of osteotomies have been attempted

about the ankle joint. Thus an osteotomy of the lower tibia realigns the ankle if it is in valgus. Osteotomies of the calcaneum to correct valgus have been tried. One of these is designed to displace the heel backwards beneath the ankle joint to provide a better mechanical advantage. These osteotomies have had limited success.

FORE-FOOT

Metatarsalgia

An interesting study was carried out by Shepherd and Vernon Roberts (1975) on 50 patients with a diagnosis of Morton's metatarsalgia—that is, metatarsalgia associated with neuroma symptoms. Analysis of the symptoms and signs revealed pain in the region of the metatarsal heads in all of them; pain radiated into the toes in 50 per cent, and toe numbness was associated with pain in 18 per cent; tenderness and swelling between the metatarsal heads was noted in all of them; divergence of the toes on either side of the affected cleft was observed in 66 per cent and reduced sensation to pin-prick in 46 per cent. At operation in all patients, flattening of the nerve was seen, but histology revealed no true neuroma formation; in 70 per cent there was an intermetatarsal bursa (figure 15.15) which was subjected to histology. Of the 50 patients, 24 per cent were diagnosed as having rheumatoid arthritis at the time of their referral and 16 per cent developed rheumatoid arthritis after referral. That is, 40 per cent of patients presenting with Morton's metatarsalgia developed rheumatoid disease. It was interesting that the diagnosis was made in 12 per cent on the histology of the excised metatarsal bursae and this was the first indication of the disease.

Metatarsophalangeal joint synovitis

Early in rheumatoid disease, synovitis of the metatarsophalangeal joints is not an uncommon concomitant of similar synovitis in the hand. If persistent and not responding to medical meas-

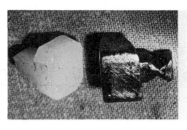
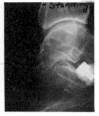

a　　　　　　　　b

Figure 15.12 (a) The valgus stop component. The metal portion is inserted into the calcaneum. (b) X-ray with prosthesis in place

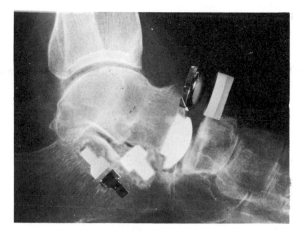

Figure 15.14 Combined talonavicular joint replacement and subtalar valgus stop prosthesis

ures, then synovectomy may be of benefit. We have carried out synovectomies on all the metatarsophalangeal joints in 18 feet: 14 continued to be symptom-free for 5 years; 4 came to further surgery within 3 years of synovectomy. Synovectomy of these joints relieves pain and seems to produce some local arrest of the disease.

GREAT TOE

The bunion or bursa medial to the first metatarsal head, in the presence of hallux valgus, is commonly involved in rheumatoid synovitis. Local symptoms can often be controlled by surgical shoes; however, fashion-conscious patients will not accept them. Despite satisfactory footwear, symptoms may progress, leading to great difficulty in walking. Surgery of 1st metatarsophalangeal joint deformities includes excision arthroplasty, prosthetic replacement and corrective osteotomies. Simple excision arthroplasties for the great toe have the disadvantage of shortening the

Figure 15.13 The talonavicular ICLH joint

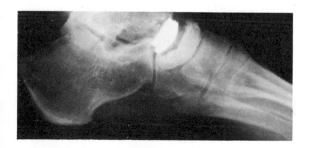

first ray and causing secondary migration of the sesamoids from under the metatarsal head to the shaft. This allows the head to drop plantarwards, thus throwing added stress on the lateral metatarsals, with consequent metatarsalgia or stress fractures of the metatarsals.

Figure 15.15 Inter-metatarsal bursa. This patient had rheumatoid disease

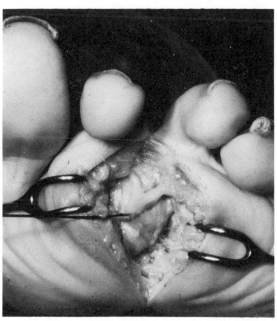

Sesamoids

Beneath the sesamoids, particularly the medial sesamoid of the great toe, there is very often a presesamoid bursa which may be involved in rheumatoid disease. Occasionally this bursa bursts through the skin, resulting in secondary infection with osteomyelitis of the sesamoid. We have excised the sesamoid for this problem on five occasions. Valgus drift of the toes is common and is analogous to ulnar deviation of the fingers. We have performed osteotomies to correct the toe valgus.

Plantar prolapse of metatarsal heads (figure 15.16)

Some operations for this problem involve excision of all the metatarsal heads—e.g., the Kates–Kessel (figure 15.17a) and Fowler (figure 15.17b) procedures. These, however, leave a floppy fore-foot with poorly functioning toes. The morbidity and immobilisation following this operation are often of an unacceptable length for rheumatoid patients, who should be kept mobile to prevent stiffness. The main indication for removing bone-stock is for an overall shortage of skin and especially if associated with ulceration. Excision must maintain the relative lengths of the respective metatarsals and often this needs X-ray control, as advocated by Kates. We have found the most satisfactory alternative procedure (Helal, 1975; figure 15.18) to be a telescoping or sliding metatarsal osteotomy at metatarsal neck level, to elevate the heads out of the fore-foot; at the same time, this produces shortening of the metatarsals and spontaneous repositioning of the metatarsal fat pad, which has generally migrated distally. The re-siting of the metatarsal fat-pad has a rewarding outcome in that the callosities disappear (figure 15.19). Temporising measures have been used in the form of metatarsal insoles to take weight off the metatarsal heads. The injection of silicone oil between the callosity and the underlying bone to create an artificial fat-pad has also been tried and is temporarily successful (Balkin, 1966). Other procedures such as insertion of silicone foam rubber between the callosity and the underlying metatarsal head have also been attempted, but

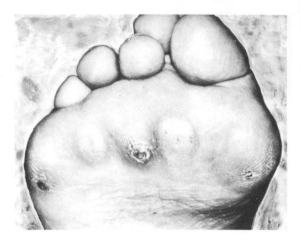

Figure 15.16 In rheumatoid disease, irrespective of the state of the joints it is always the skin callosities under the dropped metatarsal heads that give rise to the pain

unfortunately, this material tends to compress and harden, leading to recurrence (Helal, 1969). Failed excision arthroplasty of the Fowler or Kates–Kessel type, in which callosities have developed under the stumps of the necks of the metatarsals, may be salvaged by metatarsal osteotomy.

A total of 350 metatarsal osteotomies have now been carried out with a recurrence rate of callosities in 3 per cent: further osteotomies on these lead to eventual relief of symptoms. Three patients have had individual metatarsal osteotomies carried out three times. It is, of course, possible to refashion the whole fore-foot by osteotomies of all five metatarsals (chapter 5; figure 5.9). Sliding the outer metatarsal heads towards the centre of the foot helps to narrow the fore-foot and is often useful in the splayed rheumatoid foot. Osteotomy on any or all of the middle three metatarsals can be followed by immediate mobilisation with full weight-bearing, which helps to level the tread. The three middle metatarsal osteotomies can be carried out through a single incision over the middle metatarsal. If the 1st and 5th metatarsals are osteotomised, then protection of the fore-foot in a below-knee walking cast is advisable for a period

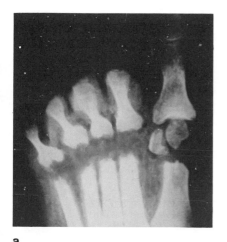

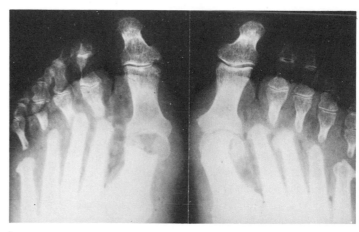

a   b

Figure 15.17 (a) Kates–Kessel operation. The desired curve has not been fully achieved. The 5th metatarsal is a little too long. The mobile sesamoids are preserved; (b) Fowler procedure. There has been a recurrence of metatarsalgia under the left middle metatarsals

Figure 15.18 Some latitude as to the site of osteotomy is permitted. The osteotomies should be done between midshaft and the neck of the metatarsal

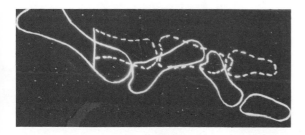

of 4 weeks. Once the acute synovitis resolves, the joints themselves rarely give rise to pain; even in the presence of subluxation of the metatarso-phalangeal joints and gross deformity of the interphalangeal joints, it is the callosity pain under the metatarsal heads which predominates. In the presence of fixed deformities associated with dropped metatarsal heads, we restrict surgery largely to the sliding metatarsal osteotomy. Because of the shortening of the ray, the deforming forces produced by the extrinsic tendons are reduced as the tendons are relatively lengthened, and very often alignment is maintained following corrective manipulations of the toes. Toe flexion deformities are manipulated to rupture the volar capsules;

Figure 15.19 Metatarsal osteotomies for dropped metatarsal heads. (a) Pre-operative. Note callosities and clawed toes. (b) Post-operative. Note narrowed foot reformation of arch, loss of callosities and unfolding of clawed toes. (c) Osteotomies at middle three metatarsal neck level. Note osteotomy of 5th metatarsal done previously for bunionette

a   b   c

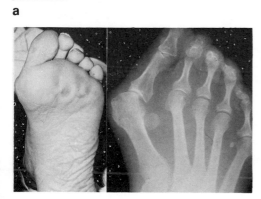

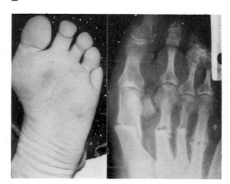

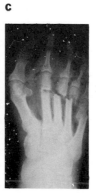

occasionally fusion of the interphalangeal joints is indicated and is aided by temporary Kirschner wire insertion if the terminal joints are to be fused. If only the proximal joints of the toes are to be fused, then Harrison–Nicolle polypropylene pegs have proved useful. Toe amputations may occasionally be necessary, but total ('Pobble': figure 15.20) excision of all toes has been rarely performed since the introduction of metatarsal osteotomy. Regnauld (1974) has employed cadaver metatarsal heads to replace those destroyed by disease. He fashions the metatarsal neck into a peg-shape upon which the correctly aligned metatarsal head is socketed. A small number of perichondrial grafts have also been attempted when only one or two metatarsophalangeal joints are involved. Early assessment suggests this may have a place in the overall surgical management.

Metatarsophalangeal joint replacement

One of the earliest implants was a Swanson proximal phalanx base prosthesis (figure 15.21). Whalley and Wenger (1978) use a Swanson finger joint, concave surface dorsally and stems in the metatarsal and proximal phalanx; they report satisfactory results. A personal series of 40 such implants confirm the findings (figure 15.22). More recently, we have used an ICLH (Imperial College London Hospital) polythene-on-stainless steel prosthesis designed by M. Tuke (figure 15.23). K. Johnson (1977), from the Mayo Clinic, Rochester, New York, describes a prosthesis in which a polythene-cupped distal component and a domed metatarsal component articulate to mimic the normal anatomy. To solve one iatrogenic problem following a Mayo arthroplasty, we have replaced the metatarsal head with a silicone rubber ulnar head prosthesis with an excellent outcome (figure 15.24). Limited experience with these prostheses is satisfactory; all can be salvaged by conversion to a pseudarthrosis.

Replacement of up to two of the lateral four metatarsal heads has been undertaken with silicone rubber finger joints; the flexion concavity is placed facing the dorsum of the foot. This procedure keeps the toes aligned, prevents excessive shortening of the affected ray and so avoids overloading of the remaining metatarsal heads.

We have frequently combined excision arthroplasty or replacement arthroplasty of the first metatarsophalangeal joint with corrective osteotomies of the lateral metatarsals to realign the toes.

Toe deformities

These are treated by formal interphalangeal joint fusions stabilised by Kirschner wires or Har-

Figure 15.20 (a) A rare intrinsic plus deformity of the toes in rheumatoid disease producing swan-neck deformity. One of the relatively few indications for (b) The 'Pobble' operation (after Edward Lear)

a

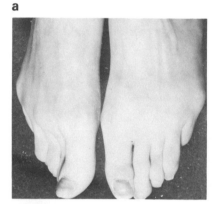

b

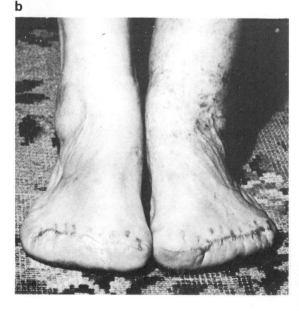

rison–Nicolle pegs. Often, manipulative correction by forcible plantar capsule rupture and Kirschner wire fixation for six weeks suffices. Gross deformities and ulceration make toe amputation the best choice. Like ulnar deviation of the fingers, lateral deviation of the toes is commonly encountered. The correction of a valgus hallux leaves the other toes in valgus. Corrective osteotomies at metatarsal neck level will allow realignment.

It must be recalled that in rheumatoid disease, perivasculitis and thromboses of vessels can occur with consequent gangrene of the toes.

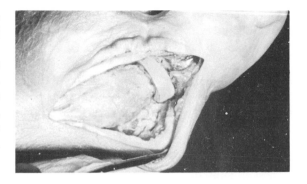

Figure 15.21 Swanson silicone rubber spacer arthroplasty of great toe metatarsophalangeal joint

THE NEUROPATHIC RHEUMATOID FOOT

Occasionally a Charcot-like destruction of the subtalar, midtarsal and fore-foot joints can occur in rheumatoid arthritis (figure 15.25). Generally, this is painless and no particular active treatment is necessary. Insoles can be provided to even the distribution of pressure on the sole of the foot. However, arthrodesis is indicated if there are high points of pressure on the weight-bearing areas of the foot.

NOTES ON OPERATIVE TECHNIQUES

Ankle joint replacement

Three approaches are in use.

Anterior approach

Through a longitudinal incision, the space lateral to the tibialis anterior tendon is developed and this tendon is retracted medially, and the extensor hallucis longus, extensor digitorum and neurovascular bundle retracted laterally. The capsule and joint are exposed. Both malleolar recesses can be seen.

Lateral approach

The skin incision overlies the fibula, which is divided 2 cm above the malleolus and pulled

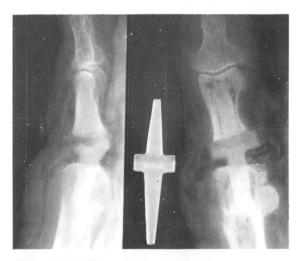

Figure 15.22 Bistemmed spacer for the great toe. This finger prosthesis is inserted with the concavity dorsalwards

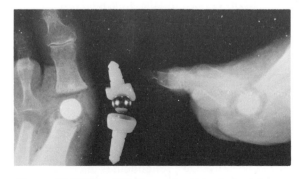

Figure 15.23 The ICLH prosthesis replacing the great toe metatarsophalangeal joint

down. The ankle is opened by hinging on the medial ligament.

Posterior approach

A vertical incision is made over the Achilles tendon, which is detached together with its bony insertion and turned cranialwards. The tendons of the medial compartment and neurovascular bundle are retracted medially. The capsule is opened and an excellent view of the joint is obtained. Subsequently the tendon insertion is re-attached by a staple or wire.

The valgus-stop operation

Positioning the foot prior to this procedure is vital. The patient's knee is flexed over the table-end and the foot rests in plantigrade fashion on a lower table or trolley so that an axial force can be put upon it by pushing down on the knee. A longitudinal incision is made just anterior to the external malleolus. The subtalar anterior facet, sinus tarsi and adjacent portion of the os calcis are exposed; holes are drilled for the stems of the talar and calcaneal portions of the prosthesis; and the appropriate spacers are inserted to separate talus from calcaneum until the heel stays in neutral, when the foot is made to 'weight-bear' by pressure on the knee. Three sizes of the polythene component of the prosthesis are available and the appropriate one is selected and cemented into place (figure 15.26).

Replacement of the talonavicular joint

This is carried out through a longitudinal incision just lateral to the tibialis anterior tendon, care being taken to avoid damage to the cutaneous branches of the anterior tibial nerve which stream down over this site. Again a special spacer is inserted. A guide is used to cut the slot for the fin on the metal talar head component. The prosthesis is cemented into place (figure 15.27).

Metatarsal osteotomies

The 1st and 5th metatarsals can be approached through individual longitudinal incisions over their dorsae. The 1st and 5th metatarsals are divided obliquely, the osteotomy slanting proxi-

mally towards the adjacent metatarsals, the metatarsal heads are displaced proximally and towards the midline of the foot (figure 5.9). The three central metatarsals can all be approached through a single longitudinal incision over the middle metatarsal. An oscillating saw is used to cut the bones just proximal to the neck of the metatarsals and the osteotomy has a 45° slant

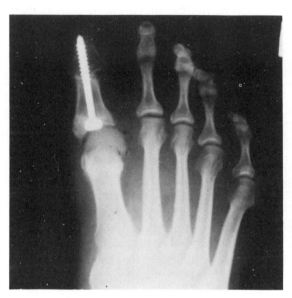

Figure 15.24 This patient has been operated on by a chiropodist. There had been an attempted arthro-desis of the interphalangeal joint combined with an excision of the metatarsal head. She was getting pain from both sites as well as metatarsalgia. Arthrodesis of the interphalangeal joint and arthroplasty of the metatarsophalangeal joint by metatarsal head replacement relieved symptoms

Figure 15.25 Rheumatoid neuropathy. These feet were painless

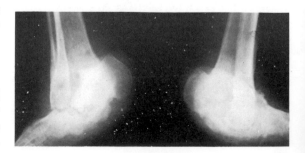

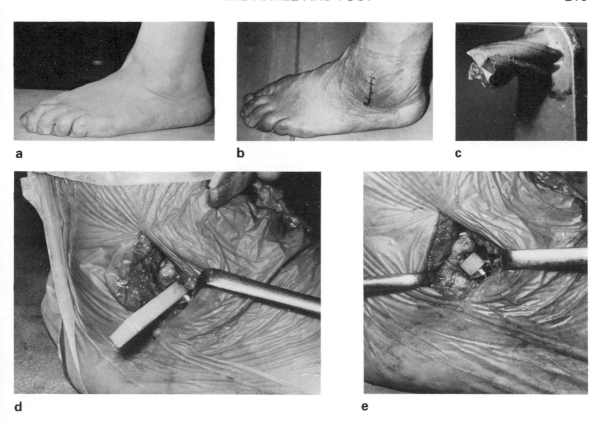

a   b   c

d   e

Figure 15.26 (a) Position of the foot for the valgus stop operation; (b) incision; (c) special reaming device; (d) spacers to gauge size of polythene component necessary to correct valgus; (e) prosthesis in place

Figure 15.27 (a) Talonavicular joint spacer. (b) Prosthesis in place

a   b

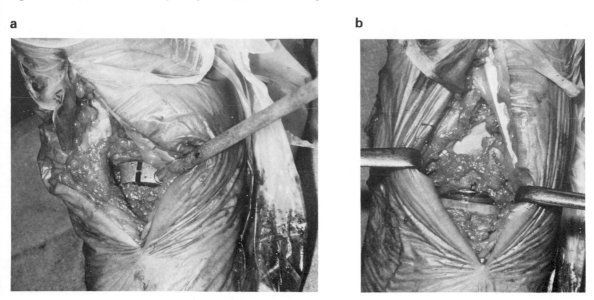

from a dorsal proximal position distally and plantarwards.

The sesamoids and plantar 'neuromata' (Morton's)

Approaches to both these should be through a longitudinal plantar incision. Incisions through the sole heal well and do not give rise to neuromata.

CONCLUSION

Although a good deal of surgical help is possible for the rheumatoid foot, the majority of patients can be dealt with conservatively by physiotherapy, chiropody and the provision of adjusted shoes and appliances. Only 10 per cent of patients come to surgery.

Implants are now available for the ankle subtalar talonavicular and metatarsophalangeal joints. All these implants are 'experimental', for none has stood the test of prolonged use. Already the designs of ankle and great toe prostheses are proliferating. In view of our limited experience with these implants, a cautious approach is advised.

REFERENCES

Balkin, S. G. (1966). Silicone injection for plantar keratoses. Preliminary report., *J. Am. Pediatr. Ass.*, **56,** 1

Buchholz, H., Engelbrecht, E. and Siegel, M. (1973). Total ankle endoprosthesis 'St Georg' model. *Chirurg*, **44,** 241–244

Fowler, A. W. (1959). The method of forefoot reconstruction. *J. Bone Jt Surg.*, **41B,** 507–513

Freeman, M. A. R. and King, J. (1975). Pain in rheumatoid hind foot. Paper read to *British Orthopaedic Foot Surgery Society Meeting.*

Freeman, M. A. R., Tuke, M. and Samuelson, K. (1975). ICLH ankle. Personal communication.

Freeman, M. A. R., Tuke, M. and Samuelson, K. (1977). Valgus stop operation. Paper read to *British Orthopaedic Foot Surgery Society Meeting.*

Helal, B. (1969). Silicones in orthopaedic surgery, *Recent Advances in Orthopaedics*, (ed. A. G. Apley) Churchill, London

Helal, B. (1975). Metatarsal osteotomy for metatarsalgia. *J. Bone Jt Surg.*, **57B,** 187–192

Johnson, K. (1977). A great toe metatarsophalangeal prosthesis. Paper read to *C.I.P. Turin*, Italy.

Kates, A., Kessel, L. and Kay, A. (1967). Arthroplasty of the forefoot. *J. Bone Jt Surg.*, **49B,** 552

Kempson, G. E., Freeman, M. A. R. and Tuke, M. A. (1975). Engineering considerations in design of an ankle joint. *Biomed. Eng.*, May, 166–180

Kirkup, J. (1974). Ankle and tarsal joints in rheumatoid arthritis. *Scand. J. Rheum.*, **3,** 50–52

Kirkup, J. (1977). Personal communication

Lord, G. and Marotte, J. H. (1973). Prosthese totale de cheville. *Rev. Chirurg. Orthoped.*, **59,** 139–151

Regnauld, B. (1974). *Techniques Chirurgicales du Pied*, Masson, Paris

Samuelson, K. (1977). The valgus stop operation. Paper read to *The British Orthopaedic Foot Surgery Society*, November

Shepherd, E. and Vernon Roberts, B. (1975). Paper read to *British Orthopaedic Foot Surgery Society.*

Whalley, R. C. and Wenger, R. (1978). Total replacement of the 1st metatarsophalangeal joint. *J. Bone Jt Surg.*, **60B**(1), 88–92

16

THE RHEUMATOID IN SOCIETY

INCIDENCE

Because there is no single universal set of criteria for the diagnosis of rheumatoid arthritis, statistical surveys differ. There are between $\frac{1}{2}$ and $1\frac{1}{2}$ million rheumatoid arthritics in the UK. Seventy per cent of these are women. In other developed countries of the temperate zone of the northern hemisphere, similar proportions of the population are affected. In the UK, 31 000 men and 104 000 women are disabled by rheumatoid arthritis and have had to give up their jobs or alter significantly their way of life (Harris, Cox and Smith, 1971). A surgeon whose patients are drawn from a population of 200 000 will have within his domain 2000–6000 rheumatoid arthritics, of which 500 will be significantly incapacitated (Lawrence, 1966; Wood, 1971). Their management is a gigantic task requiring a team of experts.

JOINT PROTECTION AND AIDS TO DAILY LIVING

Habitual positions of the limbs at rest and usual ways of handling common household articles aggravate deformity in joints damaged by rheumatoid disease. Sitting or lying with the knees and hips flexed encourages flexion contractures. Holding a handbag with the strap over the index finger increases ulnar deviation. Holding a heavy book is unnecessary (figure 16.1). Small handles of knives, forks, spoons and other implements put undue stress on the joints of the fingers and thumb. Lifting saucepans and frying-pans stresses the finger joints, which can be protected by applying the lever-arm principle when these utensils are handled (figure 16.2). Walking on hard ground with leather shoes throws unnecessary stress on the lower limb joints, and all rheumatoid patients should be advised to wear shoes with soft cellular soles and heels, which act as shock absorbers and so protect the hips and knees. This simple advice not only prevents joint damage, but also relieves pain for many years.

Slight alteration to the design of the handles of keys, knives, forks, spoons, pens and pencils (figures 16.3 and 16.4) not only protects joints, but also improves function and enables weak fingers to turn keys in locks and manipulate other common devices (Brattström, 1973). Several gadgets

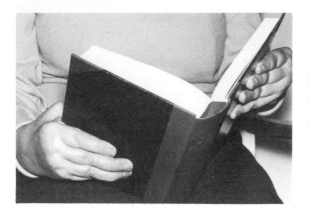

Figure 16.1 Heavy books aggravate finger deformities and are better read supported on a special rest or cushions (Brattström)

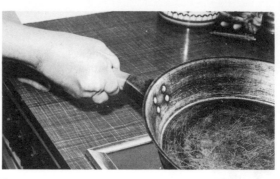

a

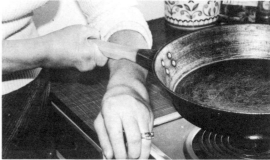

b

Figure 16.2 Lifting a heavy pan: (a) Lifting with one hand increases finger deformity and the pan is raised with difficulty; (b) using the lever arm principle, there is less stress on the fingers and the pan is easily lifted

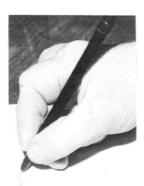

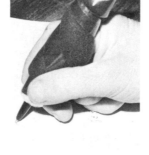

a   b

Figure 16.3 Holding a pen or pencil: (a) a narrow pen strains the fingers; (b) a simple thickening of the shaft relieves the strain

Figure 16.4 A slotted piece of wood diminishes the force necessary to turn a key

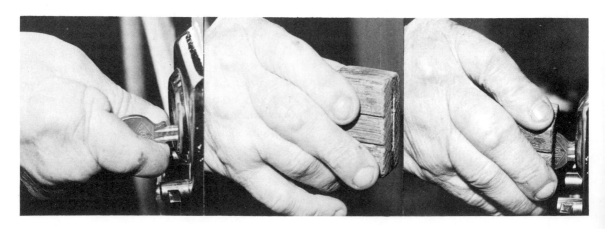

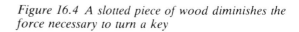

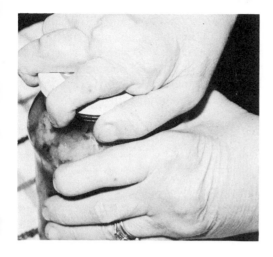

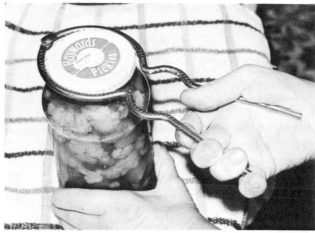

are available to assist in opening bottle and jar lids (figure 16.5) and others can be made according to the individual needs of the patient (figure 16.6).

Figure 16.5 A gadget for removing jar tops

Simple alterations in house design are helpful: rails may be fitted to walls beside stairs and toilets; toilet seats may be raised and door sills can be removed for ease of walking and wheeling chairs. Doorways should be wide enough for wheel-chairs, and steps can frequently be replaced by ramps; a simple lift is often financially feasible, although a downstairs flat is preferable.

WALKING-AIDS

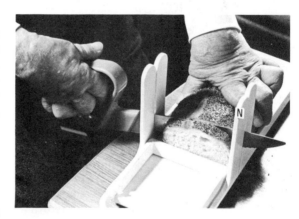

Walking-sticks, forearm crutches and quadrapod aids should be carefully adjusted to the dimensions of the patient to reduce stress on the shoulder, elbow and fingers. The handles should be large or preferably moulded from a cast of the patient's hand-grip (figures 16.7–16.9). A walking-aid not only gives mechanical support, but also increases proprioceptive sensory input, enhancing spatial awareness and improving function in a manner which is often not appreciated (figure 16.10).

Figure 16.6 A custom-made gadget for slicing bread. The handle of the knife is specially designed

standing without help. A high chair with a back rest is invaluable in the kitchen for tasks such as preparing vegetables and washing up.

WHEEL-CHAIRS

CHAIRS

Inappropriate chairs will aggravate disability, whereas a high chair or a chair with an ejector seat may offer independence, enabling sitting and

A wheel-chair in a modified house may enable a non-ambulant patient to move about and do many normal household chores from the wheelchair. A folding wheel-chair which fits the boot of the car may further extend the quality of living of a disabled patient. Wheel-chairs are available from

National Health Service sources or from the Red Cross.

DIET

The rheumatoid is frequently anaemic and may be either underweight or overweight; in either case dietary control is indicated. Rheumatoid patients tend to be in a low income group and their immobility makes it difficult for them to shop, thus aggravating malnutrition. The immobile patient who eats carbohydrates to assuage appetite becomes obese, whereas a high-protein diet suitable for such a patient is often beyond financial means (Buchanan and Chamberlain, 1977).

WORK

Physical and mental well-being is enhanced by regular productive employment, a man preferably at a place of work and a woman employed or taking the responsibility of looking after her family and household. The surgeon must encourage his patient to remain at work and, when possible, arrange the surgical regimen to make this possible. Unemployment persisting for 2 years is likely to become permanent; consequently long surgical programmes should be interspersed with periods during which the patient should return to his or her normal employment. If a patient with rheumatoid disease loses his or her job because of disability due to the disease, unemployment is then also likely to be permanent. If a return to former employment is not possible, rehabilitation should be attempted and the surgeon should be aware of local rehabilitation facilities. These include industrial rehabilitation units, government vocational training centres, sheltered workshops and the disablement resettlement officers, who may be based at the larger employment offices.

TRAVELLING TO AND FROM WORK

The difficulties of coping with public transport may prevent a rheumatoid patient travelling to and from his or her place of employment. Arrangements may be possible with fellow-workers who travel by car or a vehicle may be modified so that the disabled patient can drive but this is frequently an insurmountable problem.

SHOPPING

Inability to go shopping as a result of disability, contributes to the problem for the rheumatoid patient of retaining a place in society, and continuing normal social contacts. Management of the rheumatoid patient should enable such activities to continue if at all possible. The patient can be assisted by the physician and surgeon, not only as medical men, but also in their role as members of the community. They can use their influence in promoting modifications in the design of public buildings; many local authorities already assist the wheel-chair patient by means of ramps and wide doorways, and the picture of a wheel-chair over public conveniences so designed, is now commonplace.

RECREATION

The principles already enunciated concerning aids to daily living apply equally to recreational activities. Many arthritic patients are loath to give up pastimes such as gardening and 'do it yourself' activities in the home. Simple alterations in technique and in the devices used facilitate their handling for the disabled patients, and together with a few words of advice, can transform their lives. When kneeling or sitting on the ground is impossible, a small stool enables the patient to weed and tend plants. Spades and forks for digging are designed with a small extension which acts as a fulcrum, enabling the ground to be dug with the use of much reduced force. A small electric grass-mower is started with a switch without difficulty, whereas it is often quite impossible for a rheumatoid patient to start a petrol mower with a pull starter.

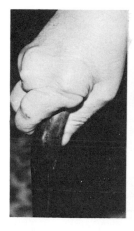
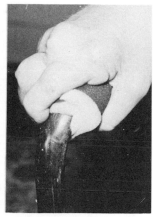

Figure 16.7 A walking-stick handle is improved by padding it

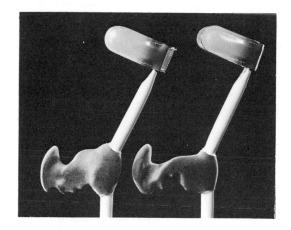

Figure 16.8 Walking aids with handles moulded to the shape of the patients hands and fingers (Brattström)

SEX

Figure 16.9 A walking aid with an integral seat and carrying basket (supplied by Doherty and Sons, Edmonton)

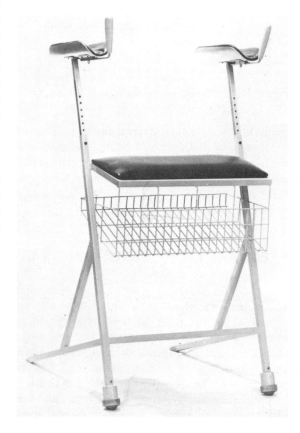

Discussion concerning the problems of sexual intercourse are seldom initiated by the rheumatoid subject in the out-patient department. If the surgeon includes this subject when taking a history, he will find that the sexual difficulties caused by rheumatoid disease may be considerable and form the basis for marital disharmony. Patients should be interviewed by a sex councillor in a quiet room adjoining the rheumatoid clinic (Greengross, 1976). Hip disease interferes with sexual intercourse (Currey, 1970; Currey and Harris, 1971); the stiff hip in the male is much less of a problem than in the female and in the latter it may make satisfactory intercourse impossible. This factor should be taken into account when deciding whether a patient should be offered a prosthetic hip replacement. For the same reason, arthrodesis of the hip should seldom be considered in the female, whereas a prosthetic hip or Girdlestone arthroplasty might be acceptable. If an intertrochanteric osteotomy is considered, it is important to know whether the sexual disability is due to pain or to limitation of hip movement. If it is due to limitation of movement, arthroplasty rather than osteotomy is indicated. When the prosthetic hip has been implanted, the surgeon should let the patient know that it is unlikely to be damaged by sexual intercourse (Greengross, 1972); however, acute hip flexion is better avoided in the first 6

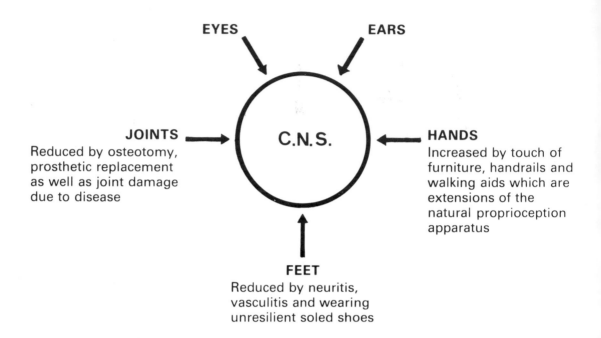

Figure 16.10 The effect of disease, joint surgery and walking aids on proprioception and so spatial awareness

weeks following total hip replacement, to diminish the danger of dislocation. Rheumatoid disease of the hands and elbows interferes with both sex play and sexual intercourse, and an understanding of this by the surgeon often enables him to relieve an otherwise unrecognised disability.

PREGNANCY, CHILDBIRTH AND BABY CARE

The surgeon's advice may be sought as to whether or not a patient is fit to become pregnant or whether an abortion and sterilisation are advisable. There are two aspects: the pregnancy and the problems of coping with an infant in its first few years of life. The only definite contra-indications to pregnancy are systemic lupus erythematosus with evidence of kidney damage, and renal amyl-

oidosis sometimes found in juvenile rheumatoid arthritis; the rheumatoid patient is otherwise capable of coping with pregnancy. She may experience a remission during pregnancy, and if there is such a remission, she must be warned that there is likely to be a relapse when the pregnancy is over, during the more difficult period when she is caring for the infant. During pregnancy most drugs should be stopped or considerably reduced, and consequently close supervision of the rheumatoid patient by both surgeon and the rheumatologist in the combined clinic is advisable during this period.

Severe hip adduction prevents the gynaecologist obtaining sufficient access for a gynaecological operation should it be necessary, but hip adduction never interferes with the actual process of childbirth and no surgical procedure on the hip joint is necessary to facilitate childbirth.

The strains, both psychological and physical, borne by a mother during the first few years of a child's life are considerable. This is the most important consideration in advising a patient whether or not to have a baby. The decision is never easy. The joy of motherhood may outweigh all other considerations. It may be difficult for the surgeon to understand that his patient may choose to put up with a degree of physical deterioration in order to have a baby. We have to accept the responsibility of giving advice when the problem may at times tax the wisdom of a Solomon.

FAMILY

The well-being of the rheumatoid patient is dependent upon proper integration into his or her own family, and the surgeon may find it difficult to realise how ignorant the layman is of many of the conditions and problems. A realisation of these problems by the family allows them a much greater understanding of the patient and this can only be achieved by education of the family as well as of the patient. This education can be started by encouraging the husband, wife or other member of the family to be present during out-patient attendances at the combined clinic. The rheumatoid patient should be treated neither as a total invalid nor as a physically normal individual, and the happy mean between these two extremes varies from one patient to another and from time to time in the same patient. The psychological interactions within a family are complex and the helpless rheumatoid, who talks of her wonderful husband doing everything for her, sometimes recovers to an extraordinary extent when her husband dies. On the other hand, it is desirable that the family be understanding of the muscular weakness and the tiredness which comes from anaemia, which is characteristic of the disease.

THE MORE DISABLED PERSON

Considerable help is now available from the family practitioner and the social services. On-going support and medication is given by the family practitioner, and social workers and trained nurses will visit the patient at home, assess problems and give practical assistance. Helpers in the home are available for housework, and regular visits by nurses can be arranged. Voluntary organisations such as the Red Cross supply wheelchairs and arrange Meals on Wheels, organisations such as St John Ambulance arrange the transport of patients from place to place and arrange regular bathing with the help of special equipment.

VACCINATION

Vaccination against smallpox is inadvisable for patients on systemic corticosteroids, because the vaccination site tends to grow in size with imperfect healing and there is also the risk of septicaemia from the infected site (Roodyn, 1977).

CONCLUSION

Orthodox medicine and surgery offer considerable relief to the majority of patients suffering from rheumatoid disease. We are seldom able to arrest the disease completely and are sometimes unable to influence its course. Rheumatoid disease encourages the practice of various branches of fringe medicines, including osteopathy, homeopathy, acupuncture, radionics, various diets and the wearing of copper bracelets. Owing to our inability to effect a cure, our patients spend time and money trying diverse remedies. We must appreciate what it is that motivates them to do this so that we will treat them with sympathy and understanding.

REFERENCES

Buchanan, J. M. and Chamberlain, M. A. (1977). Physical mobility of the disabled in Leeds. *Heberden Round.* Cardiff, May

Brattström, M. (1973). *The Principles of Joint Protection.* Student litteratur. Sweden

Currey, H. L. F. (1970). Osteoarthrosis of the hip joint and sexual activity. *Ann. Rheum. Dis.* **29,** No.5, 488–493

Currey, H. L. F. and Harris, J. (1971) *Total Hip Replacement* (Ed. M. Jayson), Sector Publishing Ltd, London, pp. 144–148

Greengross, W. (1972). *Marriage, Sex and Ar-thritis,* Arthritis and Rheumatism Council

Greengross, W. (1976). *Entitled to Love,* Malaby Press, London

Harris, A. I., Cox, E. and Smith, C. R. W. (1971). *Handicapped and Impaired in Britain,* HMSO, London

Lawrence, J. S. (1966). *Ann. Rheum. Dis.,* **25,** 425

Roodyn, L. (1977). Hospital for Tropical Diseases. Personal communication

Wood, P. H. N. (1971). Rheumatic complaints. *Br. Med. Bull.,* **27,** 1

AUTHOR INDEX

SUBJECT INDEX